GRAPHIC MEDICINE MANIFESTO

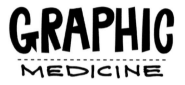

SUSAN MERRILL SQUIER AND IAN WILLIAMS, GENERAL EDITORS

Editorial Collective
MK Czerwiec (Northwestern University)
Michael J. Green (Penn State College of Medicine)
Kimberly R. Myers (Penn State College of Medicine)
Scott T. Smith (Penn State University)

Books in the Graphic Medicine series are inspired by a growing awareness of the value of comics as an important resource for communicating about a range of issues broadly termed "medical." For healthcare practitioners, patients, families, and caregivers dealing with illness and disability, graphic narrative enlightens complicated or difficult experience. For scholars in literary, cultural, and comics studies, the genre articulates a complex and powerful analysis of illness, medicine, and disability and a rethinking of the boundaries of "health." The series includes original comics from artists and non-artists alike, such as self-reflective "graphic pathographies" or comics used in medical training and education, as well as monographic studies and edited collections from scholars, practitioners, and medical educators.

graphic medicine
MANIFESTO

MK Czerwiec,

Ian Williams,

Susan Merrill Squier,

Michael J. Green,

Kimberly R. Myers,

and Scott T. Smith

THE PENNSYLVANIA STATE UNIVERSITY PRESS • UNIVERSITY PARK, PENNSYLVANIA

The panels for this volume's introduction and first page of the conclusion were drawn by MK Czerwiec and Ian Williams, based on avatars and scripts created by each author. Members of the graphic medicine community submitted the remaining panels of the conclusion.

Library of Congress Cataloging-in-Publication Data

Czerwiec, MK (MaryKay), 1967– , author.

    Graphic medicine manifesto / MK Czerwiec, Ian Williams, Susan Merrill

    Squier, Michael J. Green, Kimberly R. Myers, and Scott T. Smith.

        pages   cm — (Graphic medicine)

Summary: "Combining scholarly essays with visual narratives and a conclusion in comics form, establishes graphic medicine as a new area of scholarship. Demonstrates that graphic medicine narratives offer patients, family members, and medical caregivers new ways to negotiate the challenges of the medical experience. Discusses comics as visual rhetoric"—Provided by publisher.

Includes bibliographical references.

ISBN 978-0-271-06649-3 (pbk. : alk. paper)

1. Medicine—Caricatures and cartoons.

2. Medical care—Caricatures and cartoons.

3. Comic books, strips, etc.

I. Williams, Ian (Physician), author. II. Squier, Susan Merrill, author. III. Green, Michael J. (Michael Jay), 1961– , author. IV. Myers, Kimberly R. (Kimberly Rena), 1962– , author. V. Smith, Scott Thompson, author. VI. Title.

NC1763.M4C96 2015

610.2—dc23

2014044373

Published by The Pennsylvania State University Press,

University Park, PA 16802-1003

9 8 7 6 5 4 3

The Pennsylvania State University Press is a member of the Association of American University Presses.

It is the policy of The Pennsylvania State University Press to use acid-free paper. Publications on uncoated stock satisfy the minimum requirements of American National Standard for Information Sciences—Permanence of Paper for Printed Library Material, ANSI Z39.48–1992.

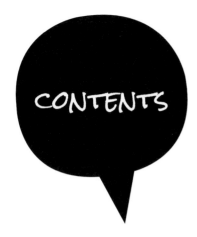

CONTENTS

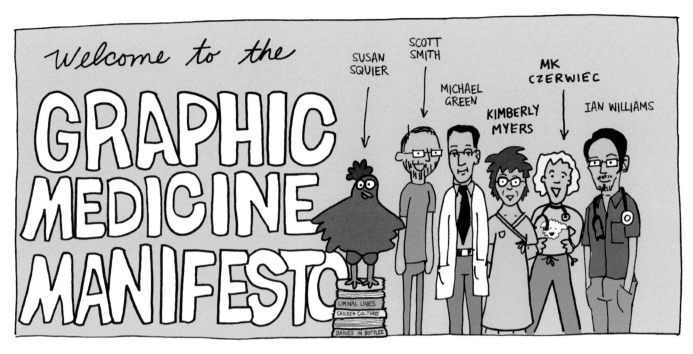

Welcome to the **GRAPHIC MEDICINE MANIFESTO**

SUSAN SQUIER

SCOTT SMITH

MICHAEL GREEN

KIMBERLY MYERS

MK CZERWIEC

IAN WILLIAMS

LIMINAL LIVES
CHICKEN CULTURE
BABIES IN BOTTLES

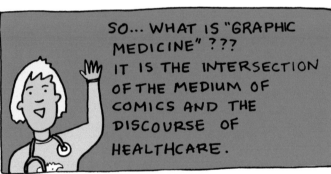

SO... WHAT IS "GRAPHIC MEDICINE"???
IT IS THE INTERSECTION OF THE MEDIUM OF COMICS AND THE DISCOURSE OF HEALTHCARE.

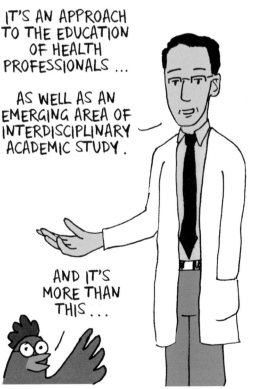

IT'S AN APPROACH TO THE EDUCATION OF HEALTH PROFESSIONALS...

AS WELL AS AN EMERGING AREA OF INTERDISCIPLINARY ACADEMIC STUDY.

AND IT'S MORE THAN THIS...

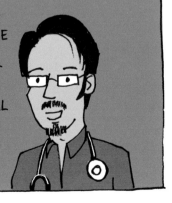

GRAPHIC MEDICINE COMBINES THE PRINCIPLES OF NARRATIVE MEDICINE WITH AN EXPLORATION OF THE VISUAL SYSTEMS OF COMIC ART, INTERROGATING THE REPRESENTATION OF PHYSICAL AND EMOTIONAL SIGNS AND SYMPTOMS WITHIN THE MEDIUM.

GRAPHIC MEDICINE IS ALSO A MOVEMENT FOR CHANGE THAT CHALLENGES THE DOMINANT METHODS OF SCHOLARSHIP IN HEALTHCARE, OFFERING A MORE INCLUSIVE PERSPECTIVE OF MEDICINE, ILLNESS, DISABILITY, CAREGIVING, AND BEING CARED FOR.

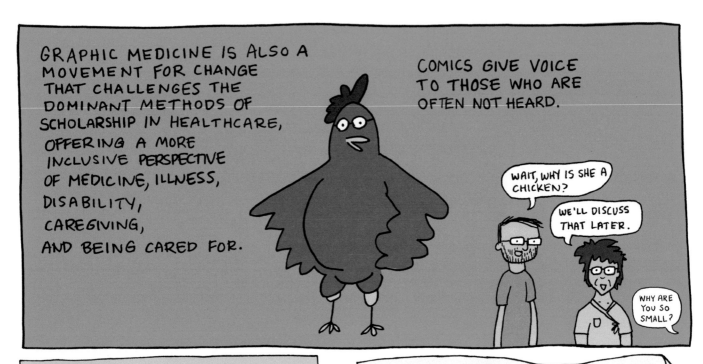

COMICS GIVE VOICE TO THOSE WHO ARE OFTEN NOT HEARD.

WAIT, WHY IS SHE A CHICKEN?

WE'LL DISCUSS THAT LATER.

WHY ARE YOU SO SMALL?

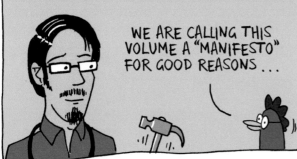

WE ARE CALLING THIS VOLUME A "MANIFESTO" FOR GOOD REASONS...

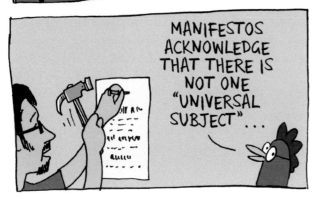

MANIFESTOS ACKNOWLEDGE THAT THERE IS NOT ONE "UNIVERSAL SUBJECT"...

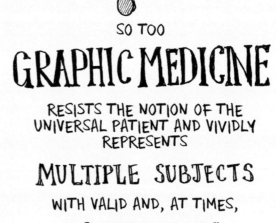

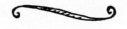

SO TOO

GRAPHIC MEDICINE

RESISTS THE NOTION OF THE UNIVERSAL PATIENT AND VIVIDLY REPRESENTS

MULTIPLE SUBJECTS

WITH VALID AND, AT TIMES,

CONFLICTING

POINTS OF VIEW AND EXPERIENCES.

graphic medicine manifesto

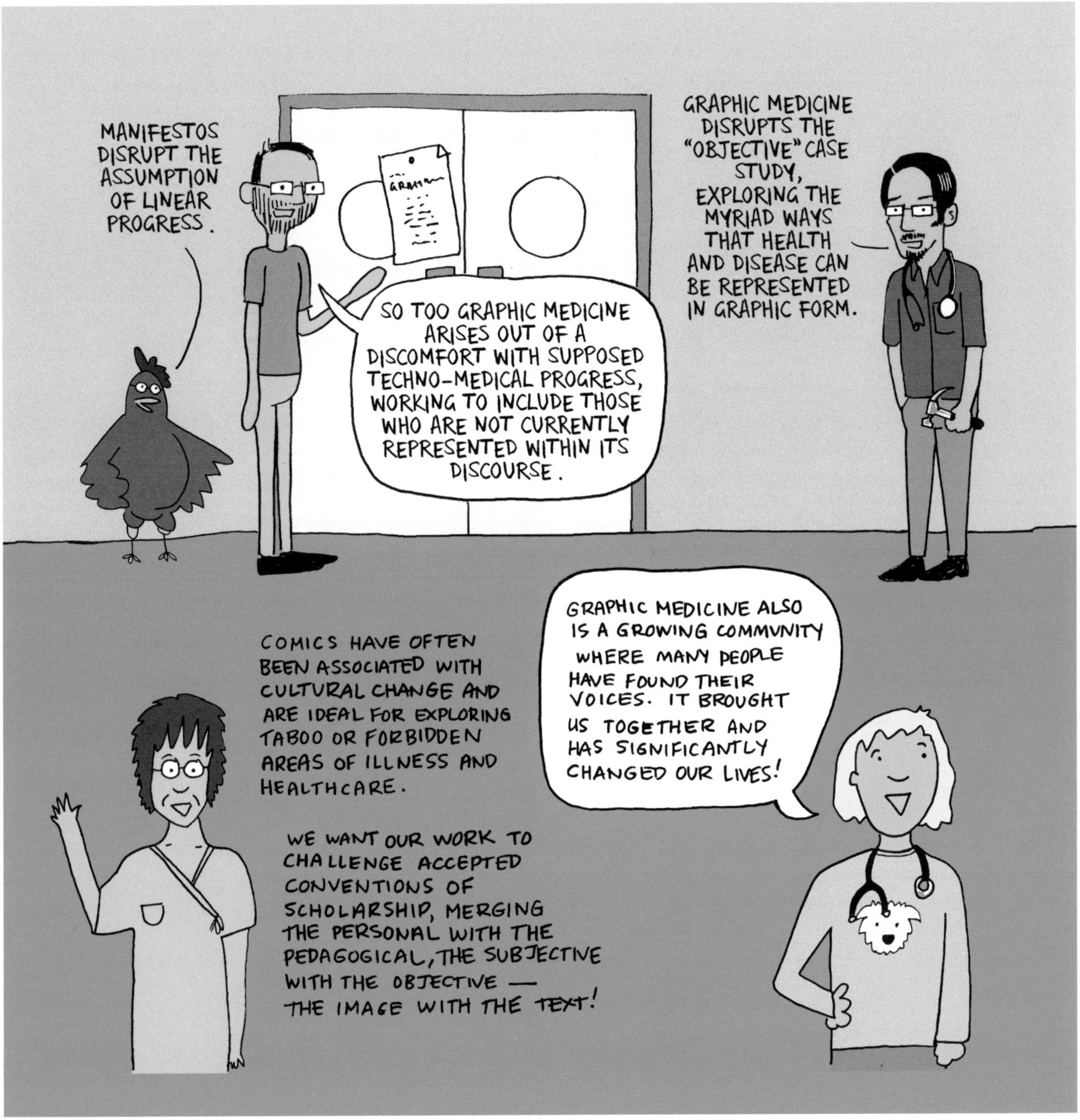
MANIFESTOS DISRUPT THE ASSUMPTION OF LINEAR PROGRESS.
SO TOO GRAPHIC MEDICINE ARISES OUT OF A DISCOMFORT WITH SUPPOSED TECHNO-MEDICAL PROGRESS, WORKING TO INCLUDE THOSE WHO ARE NOT CURRENTLY REPRESENTED WITHIN ITS DISCOURSE.
GRAPHIC MEDICINE DISRUPTS THE "OBJECTIVE" CASE STUDY, EXPLORING THE MYRIAD WAYS THAT HEALTH AND DISEASE CAN BE REPRESENTED IN GRAPHIC FORM.
COMICS HAVE OFTEN BEEN ASSOCIATED WITH CULTURAL CHANGE AND ARE IDEAL FOR EXPLORING TABOO OR FORBIDDEN AREAS OF ILLNESS AND HEALTHCARE.
WE WANT OUR WORK TO CHALLENGE ACCEPTED CONVENTIONS OF SCHOLARSHIP, MERGING THE PERSONAL WITH THE PEDAGOGICAL, THE SUBJECTIVE WITH THE OBJECTIVE — THE IMAGE WITH THE TEXT!
GRAPHIC MEDICINE ALSO IS A GROWING COMMUNITY WHERE MANY PEOPLE HAVE FOUND THEIR VOICES. IT BROUGHT US TOGETHER AND HAS SIGNIFICANTLY CHANGED OUR LIVES!

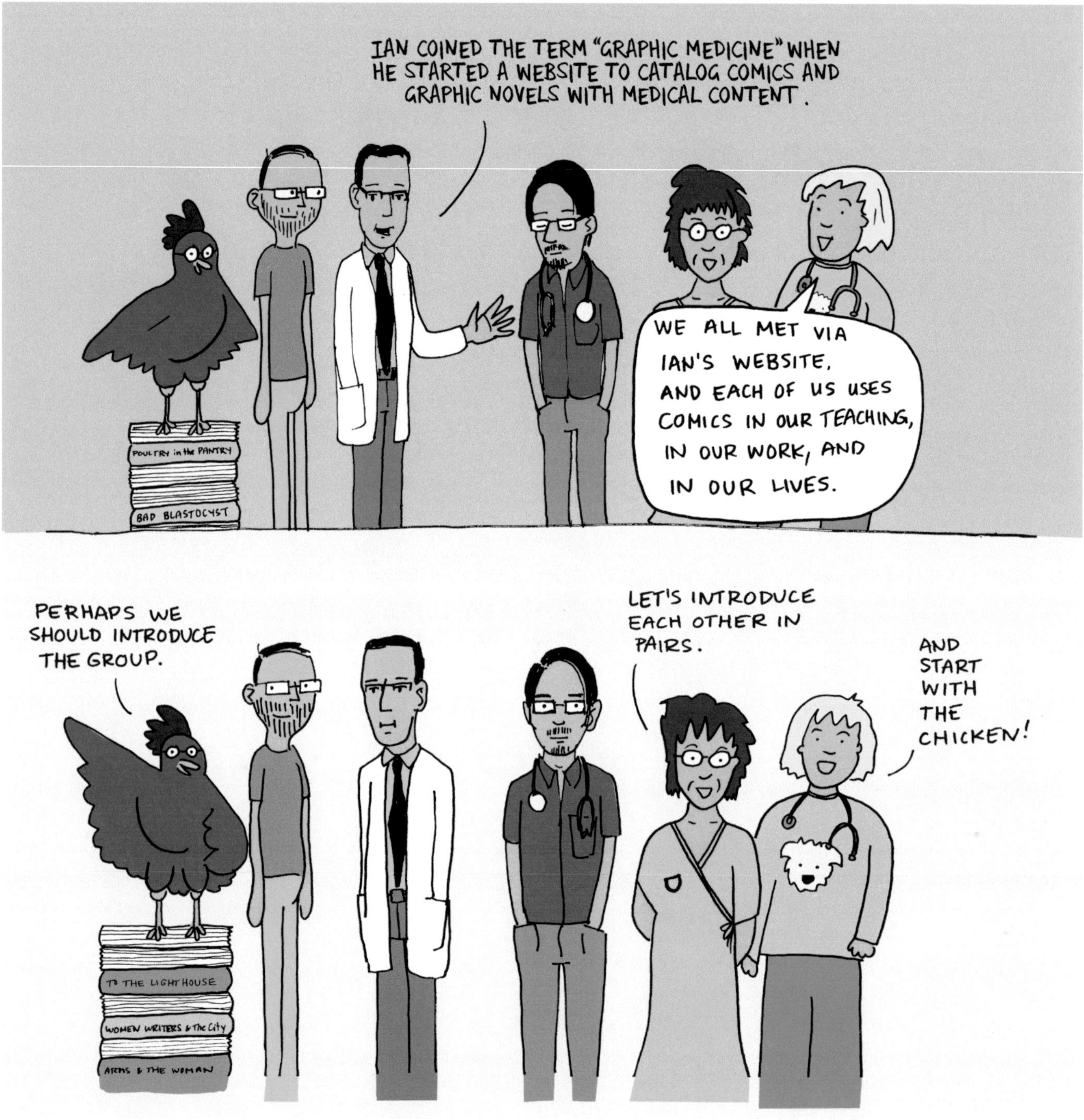
IAN COINED THE TERM "GRAPHIC MEDICINE" WHEN HE STARTED A WEBSITE TO CATALOG COMICS AND GRAPHIC NOVELS WITH MEDICAL CONTENT.
WE ALL MET VIA IAN'S WEBSITE, AND EACH OF US USES COMICS IN OUR TEACHING, IN OUR WORK, AND IN OUR LIVES.
POULTRY in the PANTRY
BAD BLASTOCYST
PERHAPS WE SHOULD INTRODUCE THE GROUP.
LET'S INTRODUCE EACH OTHER IN PAIRS.
AND START WITH THE CHICKEN!
TO THE LIGHTHOUSE
WOMEN WRITERS & The City
ARMS & THE WOMAN

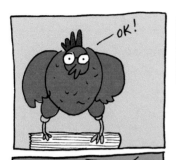

— OK!

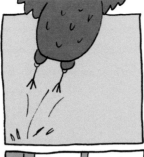

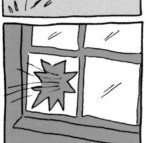

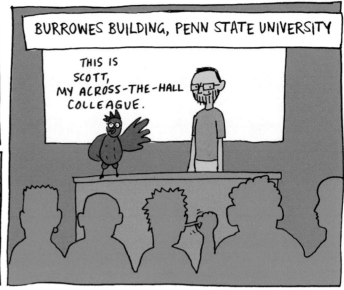

BURROWES BUILDING, PENN STATE UNIVERSITY

THIS IS SCOTT, MY ACROSS-THE-HALL COLLEAGUE.

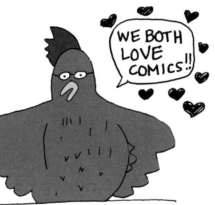

WE'VE BEEN TEACHING TOGETHER AT PENN STATE FOR SEVERAL YEARS. SCOTT TEACHES ANGLO-SAXON LITERATURE, SO I DIDN'T THINK WE'D HAVE MUCH IN COMMON. BUT THEN WE DISCOVERED

WE BOTH LOVE COMICS!!

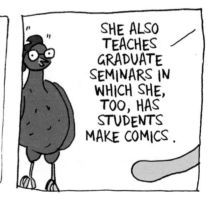

SCOTT HAS BEEN READING COMICS HIS WHOLE LIFE, TEACHING COMICS TO HIS UNDERGRADUATES, AND ENCOURAGING THEM TO MAKE COMICS TOO!

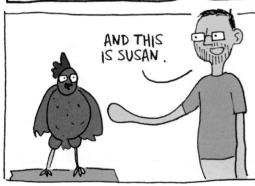

AND THIS IS SUSAN.

SHE TEACHES WOMEN'S STUDIES, MEDICAL HUMANITIES, SCIENCE STUDIES, LITERATURE... ALL IN AN INTERDISCIPLINARY WAY THAT GETS PAST TRADITIONAL FIELD DIVISIONS.

SHE ALSO TEACHES GRADUATE SEMINARS IN WHICH SHE, TOO, HAS STUDENTS MAKE COMICS.

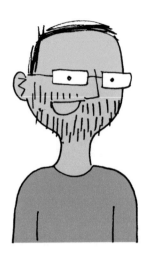

WE'VE EACH INVITED WORKING CARTOONISTS TO VISIT OUR CLASSES TO TALK ABOUT THEIR CRAFT.

WE WANT OUR STUDENTS TO EXPERIENCE THE CREATIVE PROCESS OF MAKING COMICS EVEN AS THEY STUDY THE MEDIUM.

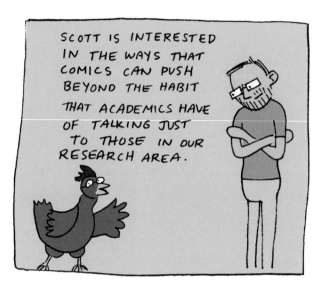

SCOTT IS INTERESTED IN THE WAYS THAT COMICS CAN PUSH BEYOND THE HABIT THAT ACADEMICS HAVE OF TALKING JUST TO THOSE IN OUR RESEARCH AREA.

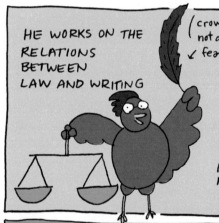

HE WORKS ON THE RELATIONS BETWEEN LAW AND WRITING

(crow quill, not a chicken feather!)

AND ON THE ISSUES OF LANDSCAPES AS PROPERTY IN THE ANGLO-SAXON AGE.

WHICH IS ALL TO SAY THAT HIS WORK IS

INTERDISCIPLINARY, socially focused,
AND CONCERNED WITH

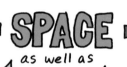

← SPACE → as well as text.

I'M INTERESTED IN HOW TEXTS WORK IN THE WORLD...

HOW PEOPLE **USE THEM** RATHER THAN CELEBRATING THEM AS MASTERWORKS.

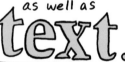

SO WITH COMICS...

I THINK ABOUT THE CREATIVE RANGE OF THE MEDIUM, AND THE DIFFERENT READING AND CREATIVE COMMUNITIES THAT ARE INTERESTED IN COMICS.

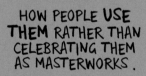

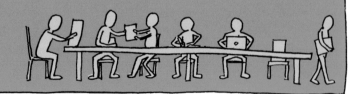

graphic medicine
manifesto

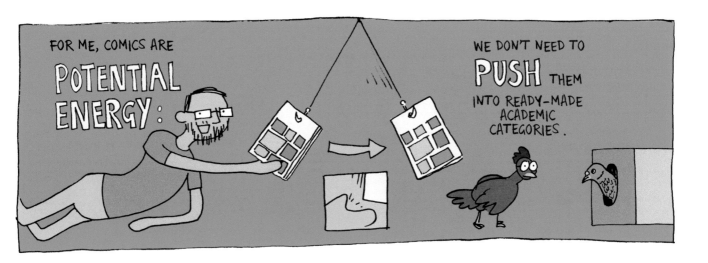

FOR ME, COMICS ARE **POTENTIAL ENERGY:**

WE DON'T NEED TO **PUSH** THEM INTO READY-MADE ACADEMIC CATEGORIES.

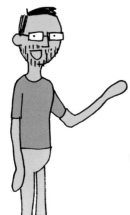

THAT'S ONE REASON I'M EXCITED ABOUT **GRAPHIC MEDICINE** – IT MEANS DIFFERENT GROUPS OF FOLKS WITH DIFFERENT INTERESTS AND BACKGROUNDS TALKING ABOUT COMICS IN **NEW WAYS.**

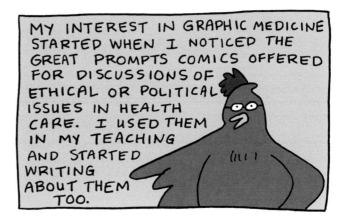

MY INTEREST IN GRAPHIC MEDICINE STARTED WHEN I NOTICED THE GREAT PROMPTS COMICS OFFERED FOR DISCUSSIONS OF ETHICAL OR POLITICAL ISSUES IN HEALTH CARE. I USED THEM IN MY TEACHING AND STARTED WRITING ABOUT THEM TOO.

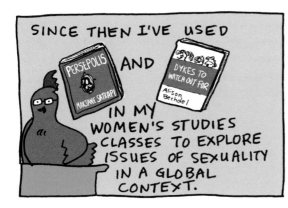

SINCE THEN I'VE USED PERSEPOLIS (MARJANE SATRAPI) AND DYKES TO WATCH OUT FOR (Alison Bechdel) IN MY WOMEN'S STUDIES CLASSES TO EXPLORE ISSUES OF SEXUALITY IN A GLOBAL CONTEXT.

AND WHEN I WORK IN ANIMAL STUDIES I'M ESPECIALLY CURIOUS ABOUT THE WAY WE SPLIT ANIMAL MEDICINE FROM HUMAN MEDICINE, SO I'VE FOUND COMICS LIKE THIS HELP ME RAISE ISSUES IN MY CLASS AS WELL AS IN MY WRITING.

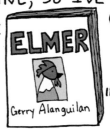

ELMER Gerry Alanguilan

(ABOUT A HEROIC CHICKEN WHO RESISTS INDUSTRIAL AGRICULTURE)

IN DISABILITY STUDIES AND THE MEDICAL HUMANITIES, THERE IS A WONDERFUL ARRAY OF COMICS TO CHOOSE FROM THAT ADDRESS ILLNESS, DISABILITY, CAREGIVING.

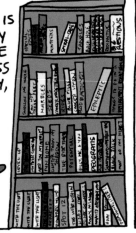

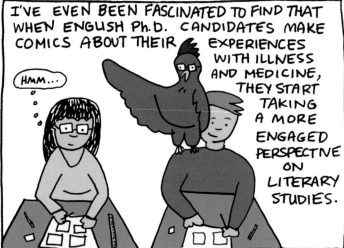

I'VE EVEN BEEN FASCINATED TO FIND THAT WHEN ENGLISH Ph.D. CANDIDATES MAKE COMICS ABOUT THEIR EXPERIENCES WITH ILLNESS AND MEDICINE, THEY START TAKING A MORE ENGAGED PERSPECTIVE ON LITERARY STUDIES.

HMM...

I THINK YOUR POINT ABOUT PERSPECTIVE IS AN IMPORTANT ONE...

COMICS ARE A POWERFUL MEDIUM FOR PRESENTING DIFFERENT WAYS OF SEEING AND THINKING ABOUT OUR VIEWS, PERCEPTION AND VALUES.

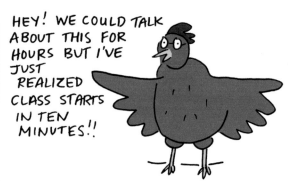

HEY! WE COULD TALK ABOUT THIS FOR HOURS BUT I'VE JUST REALIZED CLASS STARTS IN TEN MINUTES!!

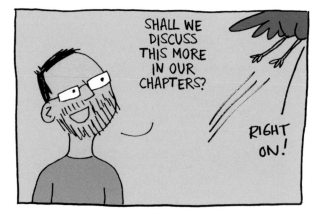

SHALL WE DISCUSS THIS MORE IN OUR CHAPTERS?

RIGHT ON!

graphic medicine
manifesto

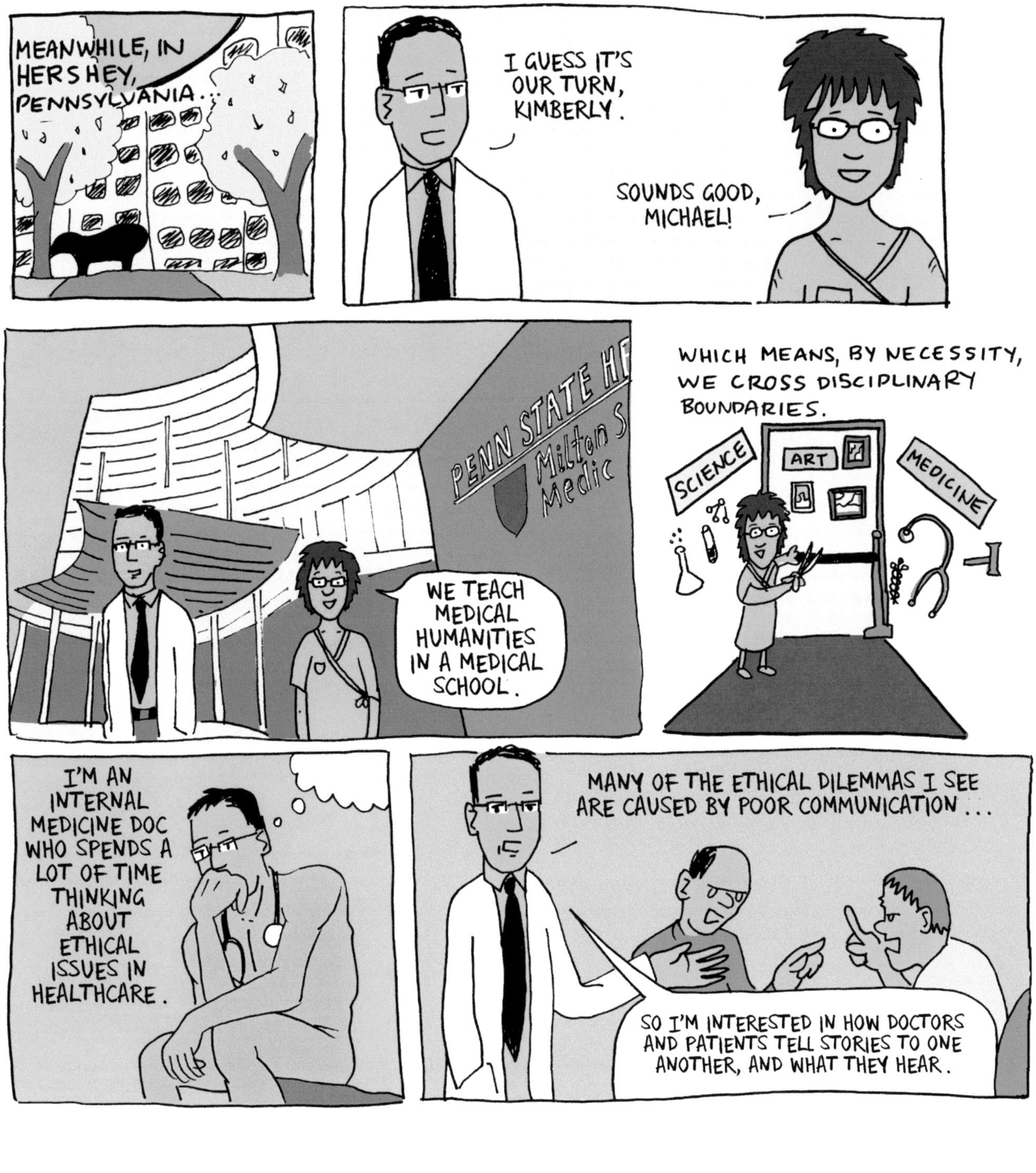
MEANWHILE, IN HERSHEY, PENNSYLVANIA...
I GUESS IT'S OUR TURN, KIMBERLY.
SOUNDS GOOD, MICHAEL!
PENN STATE HE
Milton S
Medic
WE TEACH MEDICAL HUMANITIES IN A MEDICAL SCHOOL.
WHICH MEANS, BY NECESSITY, WE CROSS DISCIPLINARY BOUNDARIES.
SCIENCE
ART
MEDICINE
I'M AN INTERNAL MEDICINE DOC WHO SPENDS A LOT OF TIME THINKING ABOUT ETHICAL ISSUES IN HEALTHCARE.
MANY OF THE ETHICAL DILEMMAS I SEE ARE CAUSED BY POOR COMMUNICATION...
SO I'M INTERESTED IN HOW DOCTORS AND PATIENTS TELL STORIES TO ONE ANOTHER, AND WHAT THEY HEAR.

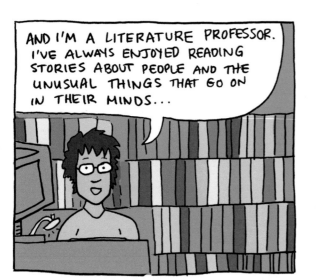

AND I'M A LITERATURE PROFESSOR. I'VE ALWAYS ENJOYED READING STORIES ABOUT PEOPLE AND THE UNUSUAL THINGS THAT GO ON IN THEIR MINDS...

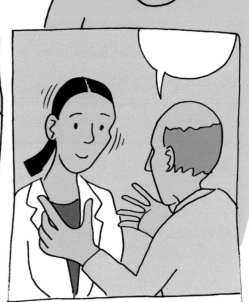

THEN, WHEN MY STEPSON GOT SICK, I BEGAN TO THINK ABOUT HOW PEOPLE'S STORIES CHANGE WHEN MAJOR ILLNESS STRIKES.

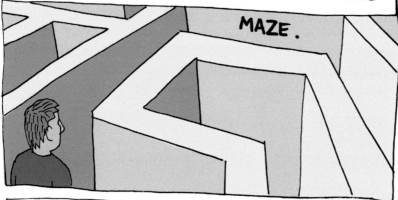

SOMETIMES PEOPLE'S STORIES GET LOST ALTOGETHER WHEN THEY BECOME PATIENTS IN A COMPLEX HEALTHCARE MAZE.

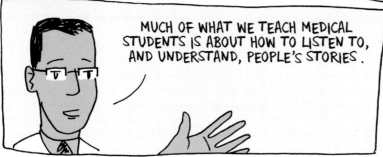

MUCH OF WHAT WE TEACH MEDICAL STUDENTS IS ABOUT HOW TO LISTEN TO, AND UNDERSTAND, PEOPLE'S STORIES.

BY FOCUSING ON PARTICULAR DETAILS, STUDENTS CAN BETTER APPRECIATE UNIVERSAL EXPERIENCES.

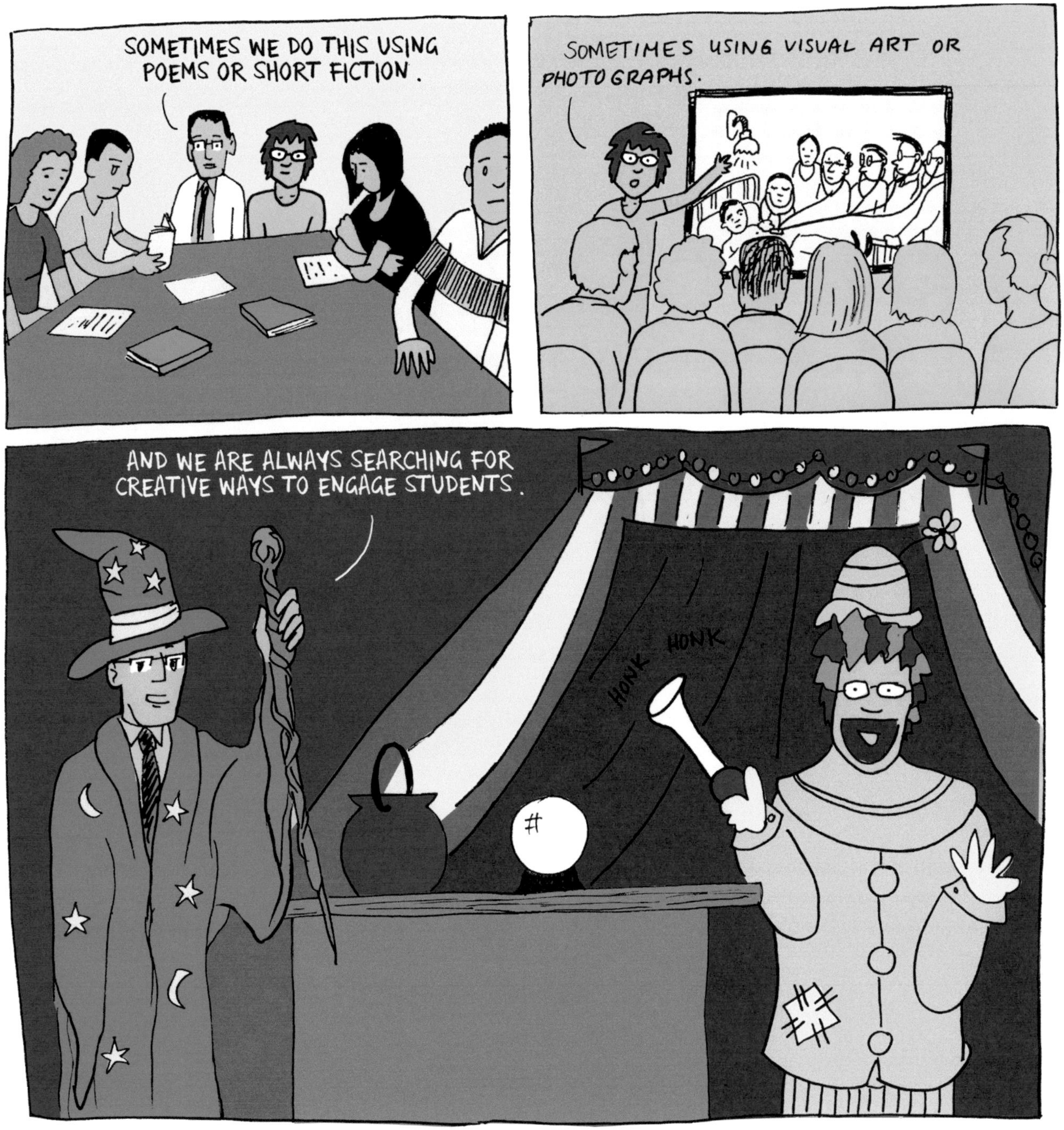
SOMETIMES WE DO THIS USING POEMS OR SHORT FICTION.
SOMETIMES USING VISUAL ART OR PHOTOGRAPHS.
AND WE ARE ALWAYS SEARCHING FOR CREATIVE WAYS TO ENGAGE STUDENTS.
HONK
HONK

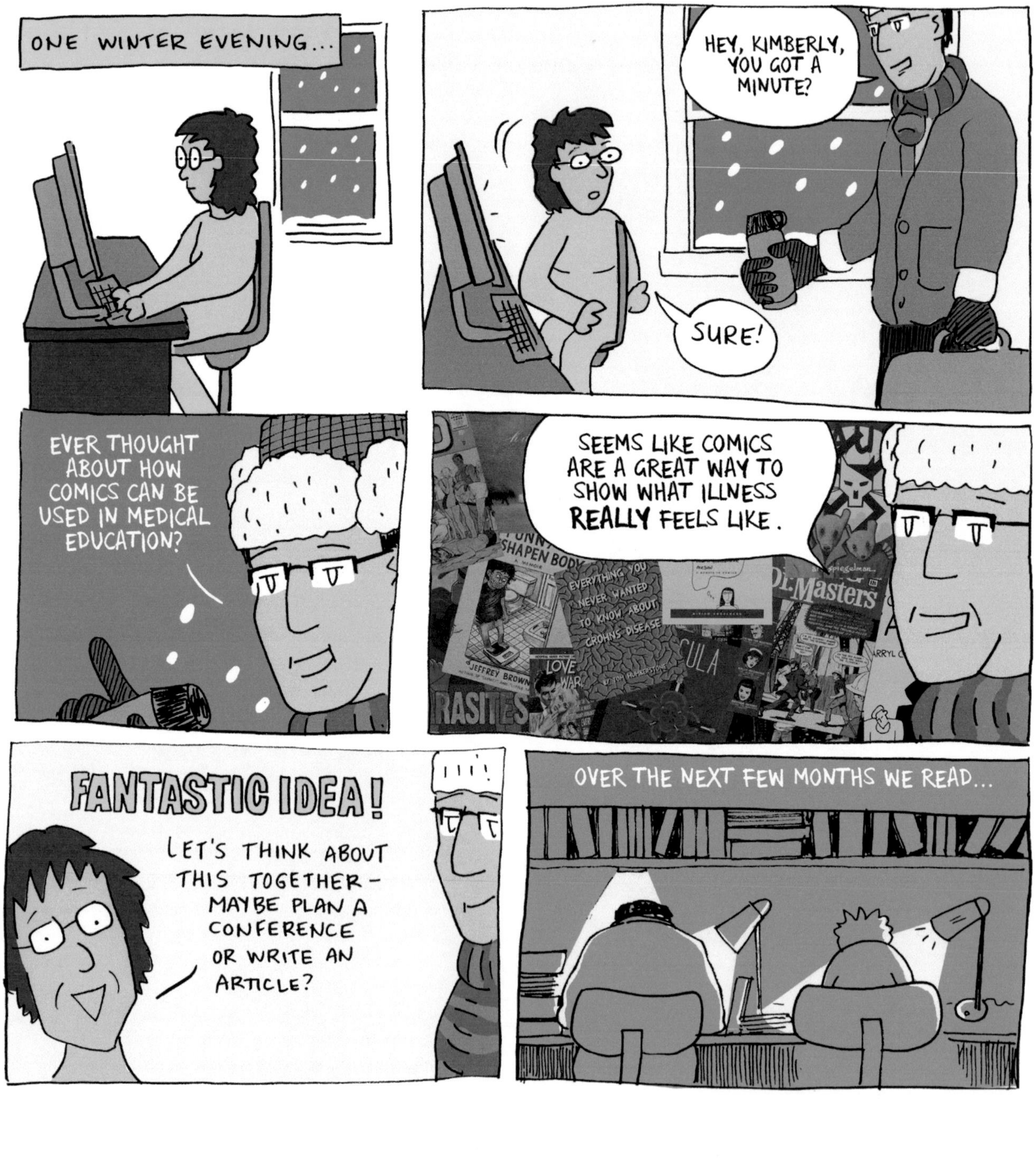
ONE WINTER EVENING...
HEY, KIMBERLY, YOU GOT A MINUTE?
SURE!
EVER THOUGHT ABOUT HOW COMICS CAN BE USED IN MEDICAL EDUCATION?
SEEMS LIKE COMICS ARE A GREAT WAY TO SHOW WHAT ILLNESS REALLY FEELS LIKE.
FANTASTIC IDEA!
LET'S THINK ABOUT THIS TOGETHER - MAYBE PLAN A CONFERENCE OR WRITE AN ARTICLE?
OVER THE NEXT FEW MONTHS WE READ...

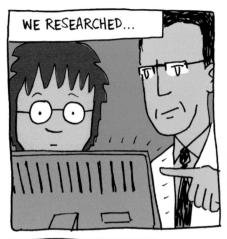

WE RESEARCHED...

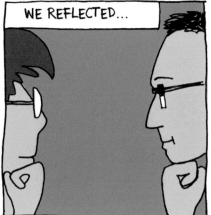

WE REFLECTED...

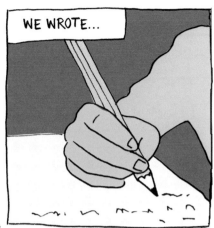

WE WROTE...

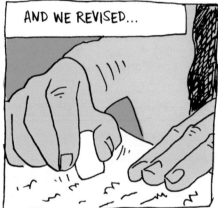

AND WE REVISED...

UNTIL WE PUBLISHED A

LANDMARK

ARTICLE ABOUT THE USE OF COMICS IN MEDICAL EDUCATION.

IT WAS THE FIRST OVERVIEW OF COMICS IN MEDICINE IN A

MAJOR MEDICAL JOURNAL!

WE EVEN MADE THE COVER!

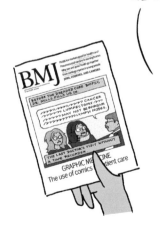

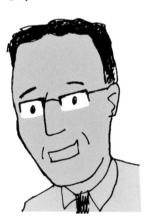

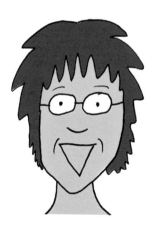

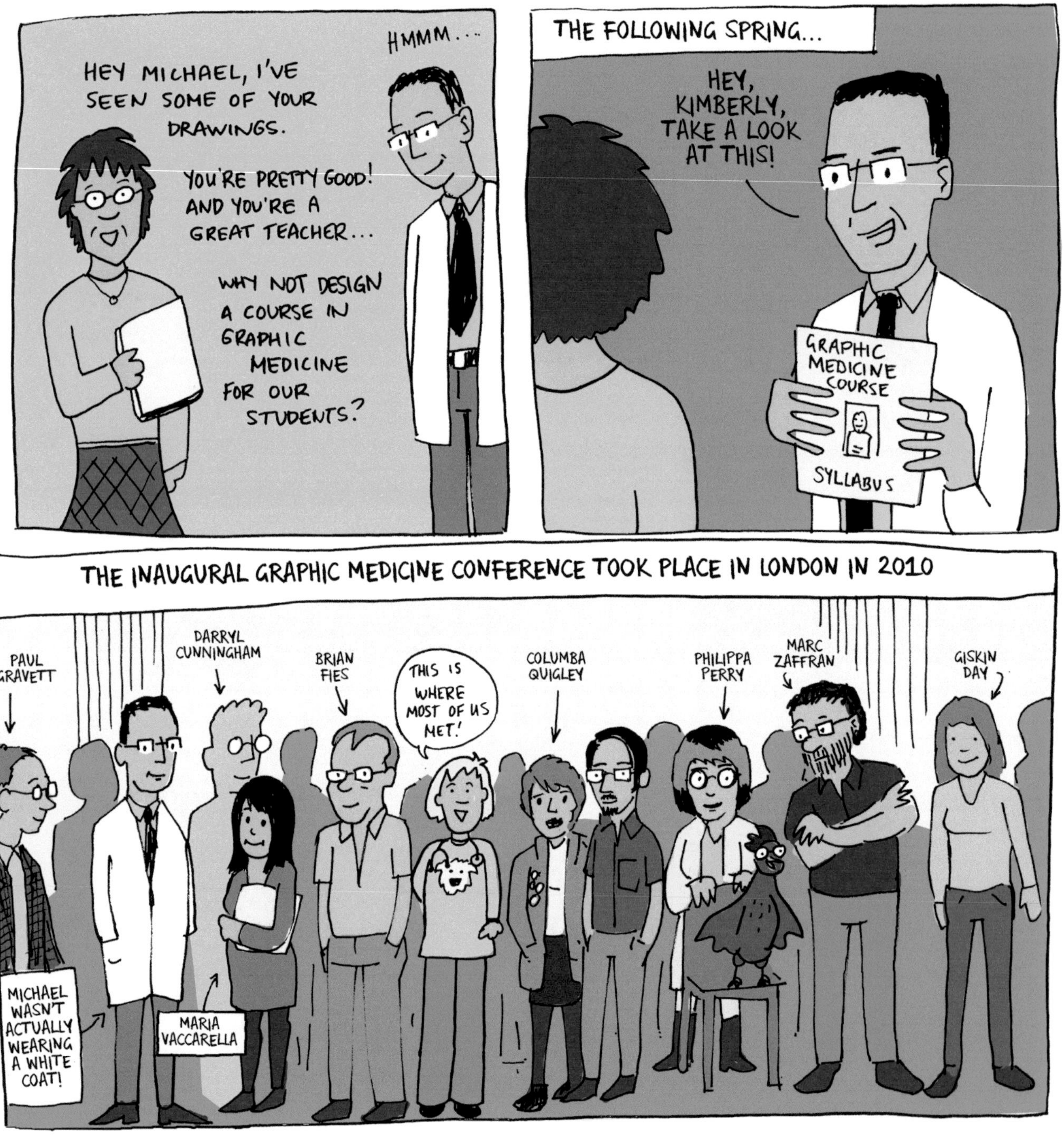
HEY MICHAEL, I'VE SEEN SOME OF YOUR DRAWINGS.
YOU'RE PRETTY GOOD! AND YOU'RE A GREAT TEACHER...
WHY NOT DESIGN A COURSE IN GRAPHIC MEDICINE FOR OUR STUDENTS?
HMMM...
THE FOLLOWING SPRING...
HEY, KIMBERLY, TAKE A LOOK AT THIS!
GRAPHIC MEDICINE COURSE
SYLLABUS
THE INAUGURAL GRAPHIC MEDICINE CONFERENCE TOOK PLACE IN LONDON IN 2010
PAUL GRAVETT
DARRYL CUNNINGHAM
BRIAN FIES
THIS IS WHERE MOST OF US MET!
COLUMBA QUIGLEY
PHILIPPA PERRY
MARC ZAFFRAN
GISKIN DAY
MICHAEL WASN'T ACTUALLY WEARING A WHITE COAT!
MARIA VACCARELLA

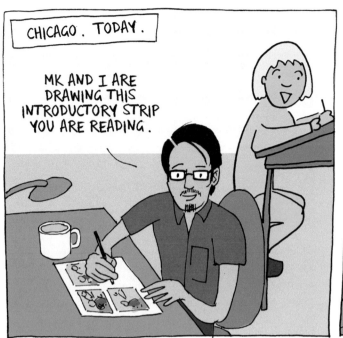

CHICAGO. TODAY.

MK AND I ARE DRAWING THIS INTRODUCTORY STRIP YOU ARE READING.

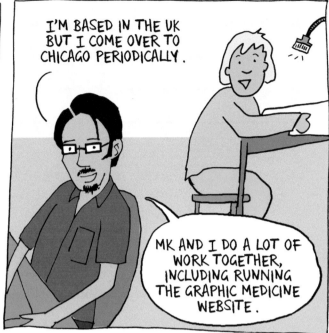

I'M BASED IN THE UK BUT I COME OVER TO CHICAGO PERIODICALLY.

MK AND I DO A LOT OF WORK TOGETHER, INCLUDING RUNNING THE GRAPHIC MEDICINE WEBSITE.

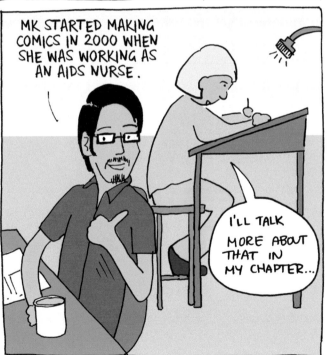

MK STARTED MAKING COMICS IN 2000 WHEN SHE WAS WORKING AS AN AIDS NURSE.

I'LL TALK MORE ABOUT THAT IN MY CHAPTER...

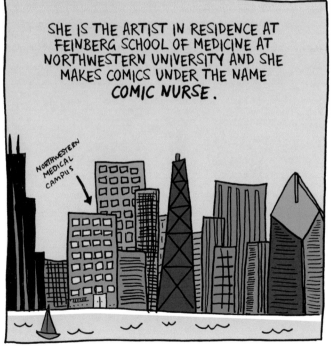

SHE IS THE ARTIST IN RESIDENCE AT FEINBERG SCHOOL OF MEDICINE AT NORTHWESTERN UNIVERSITY AND SHE MAKES COMICS UNDER THE NAME COMIC NURSE.

NORTHWESTERN MEDICAL CAMPUS

BY COINCIDENCE BOTH IAN AND I DID MASTER'S DEGREES IN MEDICAL HUMANITIES, WHERE WE FOCUSED ON MEDICAL STORIES IN COMICS.

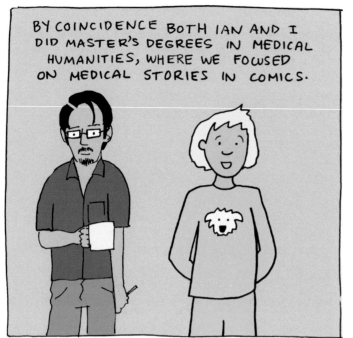

IAN IS A PHYSICIAN AND COMICS ARTIST.

HE SET UP THE GRAPHIC MEDICINE WEBSITE IN 2007 AND WAS THE MAIN ORGANIZER OF THE FIRST CONFERENCE IN 2010, IN LONDON.

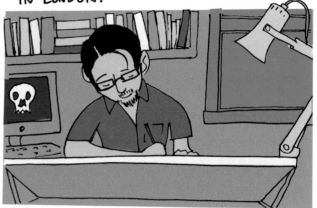

AND I COORDINATED THE SECOND CONFERENCE IN CHICAGO A YEAR LATER. SINCE THEN, ANNUAL "COMICS & MEDICINE" CONFERENCES HAVE BROUGHT TOGETHER PEOPLE FROM ALL OVER THE WORLD WHO DO THIS WORK.

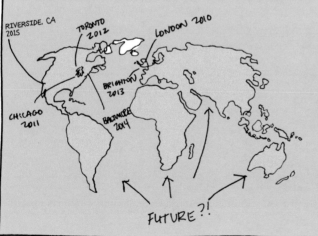

SINCE 2011 GRAPHIC MEDICINE HAS PRACTICALLY BECOME OUR FULL-TIME WORK.

LIKE OUR COLLEAGUES, WE TEACH AND WRITE ABOUT THE SUBJECT, GETTING PEOPLE TO DRAW COMICS AS A WAY OF THINKING ABOUT HEALTH CARE AND THEIR EXPERIENCES IN IT.

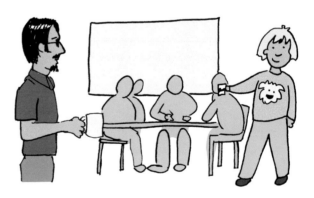

graphic medicine manifesto

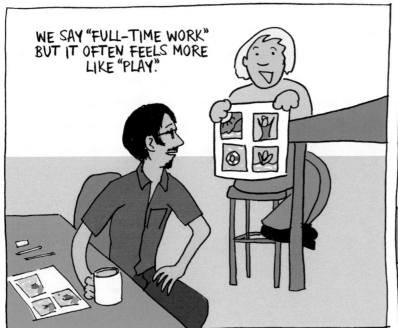

WE SAY "FULL-TIME WORK" BUT IT OFTEN FEELS MORE LIKE "PLAY."

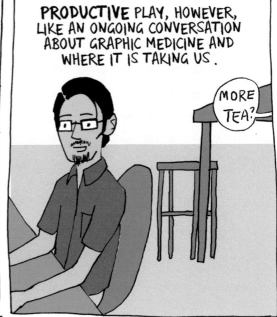

PRODUCTIVE PLAY, HOWEVER, LIKE AN ONGOING CONVERSATION ABOUT GRAPHIC MEDICINE AND WHERE IT IS TAKING US.

MORE TEA?

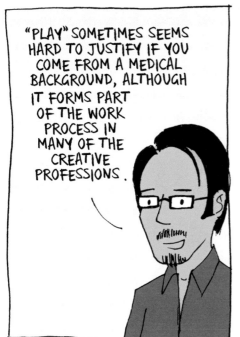

"PLAY" SOMETIMES SEEMS HARD TO JUSTIFY IF YOU COME FROM A MEDICAL BACKGROUND, ALTHOUGH IT FORMS PART OF THE WORK PROCESS IN MANY OF THE CREATIVE PROFESSIONS.

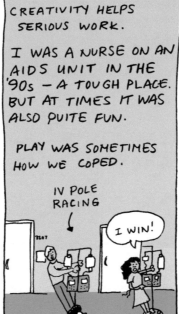

CREATIVITY HELPS SERIOUS WORK.

I WAS A NURSE ON AN AIDS UNIT IN THE '90s — A TOUGH PLACE. BUT AT TIMES IT WAS ALSO QUITE FUN.

PLAY WAS SOMETIMES HOW WE COPED.

IV POLE RACING

I WIN!

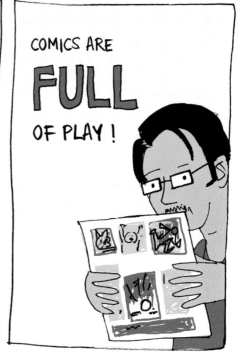

COMICS ARE

FULL

OF PLAY!

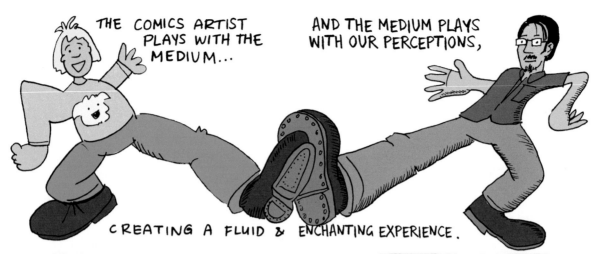

THE COMICS ARTIST PLAYS WITH THE MEDIUM...

AND THE MEDIUM PLAYS WITH OUR PERCEPTIONS,

CREATING A FLUID & ENCHANTING EXPERIENCE.

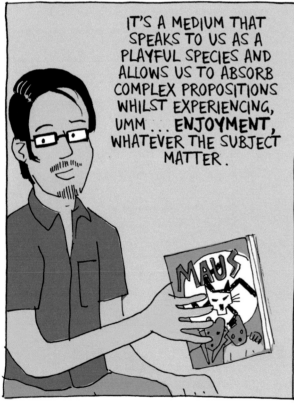

IT'S A MEDIUM THAT SPEAKS TO US AS A PLAYFUL SPECIES AND ALLOWS US TO ABSORB COMPLEX PROPOSITIONS WHILST EXPERIENCING, UMM ... **ENJOYMENT,** WHATEVER THE SUBJECT MATTER.

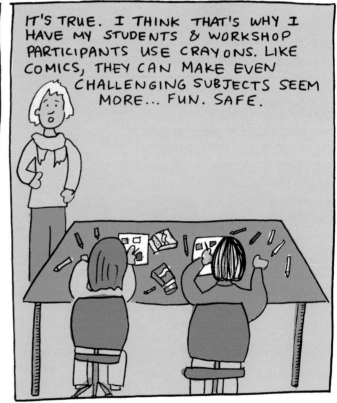

IT'S TRUE. I THINK THAT'S WHY I HAVE MY STUDENTS & WORKSHOP PARTICIPANTS USE CRAYONS. LIKE COMICS, THEY CAN MAKE EVEN CHALLENGING SUBJECTS SEEM MORE... FUN. SAFE.

graphic medicine
manifesto

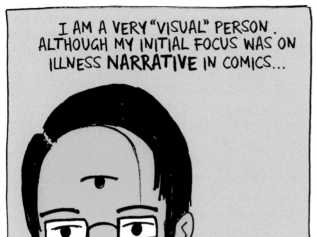

I AM A VERY "VISUAL" PERSON. ALTHOUGH MY INITIAL FOCUS WAS ON ILLNESS **NARRATIVE** IN COMICS...

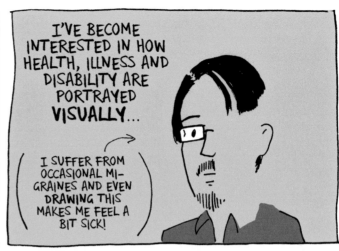

I'VE BECOME INTERESTED IN HOW HEALTH, ILLNESS AND DISABILITY ARE PORTRAYED **VISUALLY**...

I SUFFER FROM OCCASIONAL MI-GRAINES AND EVEN DRAWING THIS MAKES ME FEEL A BIT SICK!

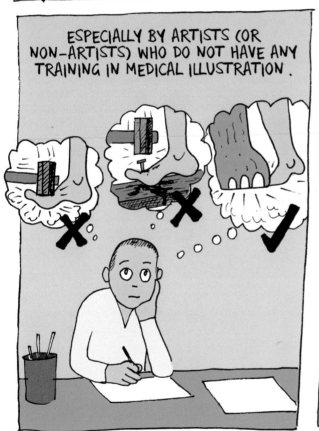

ESPECIALLY BY ARTISTS (OR NON-ARTISTS) WHO DO NOT HAVE ANY TRAINING IN MEDICAL ILLUSTRATION.

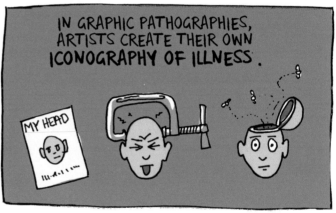

IN GRAPHIC PATHOGRAPHIES, ARTISTS CREATE THEIR OWN **ICONOGRAPHY OF ILLNESS**.

MY HEAD

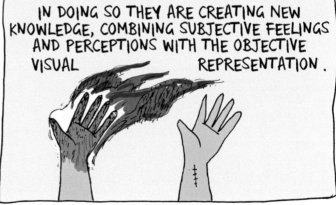

IN DOING SO THEY ARE CREATING NEW KNOWLEDGE, COMBINING SUBJECTIVE FEELINGS AND PERCEPTIONS WITH THE OBJECTIVE VISUAL REPRESENTATION.

THIS WAS TRADITIONALLY THE DOMAIN OF THE DOCTOR OR MEDICAL ARTIST WHO WIELDED POWER BY CONTROLLING AND STANDARDIZING THE WAY THAT DISEASES WERE VISUALIZED.

MORE LIVID, MAN!

GRAPHIC MEDICINE SEEKS TO DISRUPT THIS POWER IMBALANCE! WE BELIEVE THOSE BEST POSITIONED TO REPRESENT ILLNESS AND CARE-GIVING ARE THOSE LIVING WITH IT.

NIHIL DE NOBIS, SINE NOBIS!

EACH AUTHOR IN THIS MANIFESTO BRINGS A UNIQUE PERSPECTIVE TO GRAPHIC MEDICINE.

IN THE FOLLOWING CHAPTERS, EACH OF US EXPANDS OUR VIEW.

AND SHARES AN EXAMPLE OF GRAPHIC MEDICINE AT WORK.

SO LET'S GET STARTED!

ALTHOUGH THERE ARE OTHERS TO BE EXPLORED.

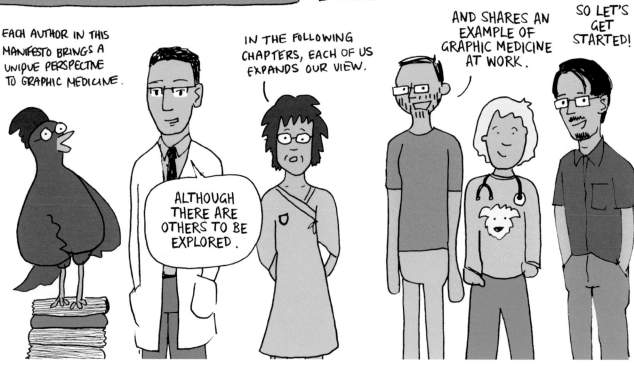

graphic medicine
manifesto

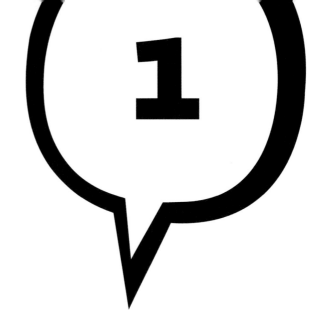

Who Gets to Speak?

The Making of Comics Scholarship

— — — — —

Scott T. Smith

My earliest reading memories are of comics. As I grew up in the rural Midwest during the 1970s and 1980s, comics were available to me in limited and often unpredictable ways. The local drugstore carried some mainstream comics, as did the local grocery (along with a few edgier black-and-white magazines like *Cracked* or *The Savage Sword of Conan*), but there was no bookstore and certainly no specialty comics shop in our small town of 800 people. But there were yard sales. Long before the days of the collector market and eBay, people were quite happy to sell off their old comics for next to nothing. One of my uncles might stop by our house and drop off a few grocery bags of old comics he had picked up on the cheap at an estate auction, or I might manage to hit the annual yard sale of a local collector before the other kids got wise, hauling home a pile of four-color treasures with giddy joy. In such ways, I accumulated a makeshift collection of comics, which, when combined with the substantial holdings my friend Eric had inherited from his older brother and sisters, made up a scattershot archive of mainstream comics that reached back into the 1960s. Certain titles and runs from our shared hoard are forever burned into my memory: Steve Gerber's iconoclastic *Howard the Duck*, Chris Claremont and John Byrne's famed *X-Men* run, a handful of bizarre *Weird War Tales* comics, Frank Miller's noir-with-ninjas *Daredevil*, and the hokey-but-always-cool Legion of Super-Heroes from the 1960s *Adventure Comics*.

I also unearthed a stash of forgotten comics tucked away in my Grandma Jean's house, consisting of older titles from Marvel, Charleston,

Gold Key, and Classics Illustrated. She also had a copy of the oversized *Smithsonian Collection of Newspaper Comics*, which reprinted early strips like *The Katzenjammer Kids* and *Little Nemo in Slumberland*. These classic newspaper comics amazed me with their scale and ambition—all this material together made me think that comics could do anything, be about anything. What strikes me now about this patchwork archive is how utterly random it was. I read what I could find locally, much of it older comics, supplemented by whatever occasional new titles I might pick up at a nearby store or through an occasional mail subscription. And aside from a very few collections in book form, I read comics as individual issues.

These reading experiences gave me an abiding appreciation of comics as a popular medium with a long and rich history. At the same time, I was completely unaware of underground and alternative comics—there were simply no venues for their distribution in rural Missouri (or at least none that I was aware of at the time). My interest in comics took a turn after 1986, though, when I was old enough to drive to a recently opened comic shop about forty miles from my hometown. In this modest little store, run by a teenage entrepreneur out of his family garage, I encountered comics that were then driving innovation in the mainstream: Frank Miller's *The Dark Knight Returns*, Alan Moore and Dave Gibbons's *Watchmen*, Frank Miller and Bill Sienkiewicz's *Elektra: Assassin*, and J. M. DeMatteis and Jon Muth's *Moonshadow* (none of which had been published under the content restrictions of the Comics Code Authority). These comics were all doing something new, and they all felt groundbreaking in some way. Suddenly the medium looked very different.

After I went to college a few years later, my interest in comics began to wane, largely due to fatigue with the superhero genre. If I had lived in a larger city, perhaps, I might have found comics like Paul Chadwick's *Concrete* or the Hernandez brothers' *Love and Rockets* to provide an alternative to the bloated mainstream, which had largely transformed into a collector's market that would soon prove fatal to many publishers and comic shops. By my junior year, I had pretty much given up on comics and taken up with the literary fiction fashionable among earnest English majors. I would occasionally dip back into comics—drawn to titles like Neil Gaiman's literary-baroque *Sandman* or Garth Ennis and Steve Dillon's grossly irreverent *Preacher*—but I wouldn't read them again on a regular basis until I returned to graduate school in the early 2000s.

My interest in comics was reignited when I was working through a rigorous English doctoral program with a focus on Anglo-Saxon language and literature. My return to comics coincided with my return to the university, and this convergence has undoubtedly shaped my thinking on the medium and its scholarship. At that time, I also found a public library with a substantial collection of comics and graphic novels as well as two local comic shops that carried more mainstream fare. For the first time I had easy access to a wide variety of comics new and old, alternative and mainstream.

Comics at first provided an anodyne for the grind of graduate school, but I soon began to think about the possibilities of comics criticism within an academic environment. I read whatever scholarship I could find on comics, even as I went through blogs and other online forums on a regular basis. I was struck by two things. One, it seemed that scholars weren't yet sure what to say about comics or how they should go about saying it—in part due to the lack of an established scholarly tradition on comics. (This was in stark contrast to my experience with other areas of literary study, especially medieval literature, which had generated a vast field of secondary scholarship and resources.) Two, much of what I read by nonacademics was more insightful, informed, and rhetorically effective than what I was reading in university press publications and professional journals. It seemed to me at the time that the academy was running behind. Things have certainly changed over the last decade, as comics studies has become charged with an energy and open potential that seem entirely uncommon in academic disciplines. But part of that energy has come from comics criticism's prehistory.

This past life in the public sphere, prior to and largely outside of academic discourse, makes comics studies especially exciting as a field that has the capacity to include and speak to diverse communities. Comics studies has the real potential to produce a public and open criticism that is responsive and accessible to both specialists and nonspecialists, to creators and critics, to casual readers and aficionados, to academics and nonacademics alike. Currently, comics criticism is quite strong outside the academy, as a number of writers and creators regularly produce quality work across a number of venues. Academic writing on comics stands to benefit from the contributions of those outside the university by engaging in an open conversation that welcomes and values many voices and perspectives.

Academic writing on comics has itself gained steady momentum and mass since the early 1990s. The last decade, especially, witnessed a flurry of academic publishing and activity interested in or featuring comics. Indeed, comics studies looks very much like a genuine growth area in academic scholarship.[1] A number of online and print journals are now dedicated to or include work on comics, for example, while both university and popular presses have issued new and reprint titles in a competitive rush.[2] Comics have likewise gained more presence in university classrooms and libraries, a development that demonstrates a growing level of institutional interest and support among teachers, librarians, and administrators. At the same time, comics scholarship remains an emerging field currently engaged in the ongoing (and occasionally tortuous) process of its own self-definition and delineation. Charles Hatfield has recently noted that "much of the work that goes on in a new field involves trying to define it. Academic comics study, not exactly a new but certainly a newly self-conscious field, has been particularly notable for this sort of anxious throat-clearing."[3] As Hatfield suggests, much current scholarship seems preoccupied with establishing definitions and justifying comics studies as a legitimate area of academic work. The time and need for this defensive reflex, though, has largely passed—comics studies no longer needs to apologize for its subject matter. In Greg M. Smith's opinion, "For Comics Studies to mature as a field, academics need to assert they can study comics (as complex texts, as industrially produced objects, as culture in circulation) without making excuses for their devalued status. My suggestion would be to do solid, complex scholarly work on comics without apology, work that undisputedly provides insight. If we act as if we don't need to justify our place, then the work itself will be its most powerful justification."[4] Unfortunately, through a lingering commitment to apology and self-justification, academic writing on comics has fallen into a number of habits and assumptions that keep the field in a prolonged moment of self-identification and self-defense.

This essay aims first to assess the current state and status of comics studies, with a particular focus on English-language comics and scholarship, followed by some suggestions on how the field might move forward in productive ways, especially as a discipline that is not primarily confined to (or claimed by) academic departments of literature.

Comics, Criticism, and the Academy

What follows is an overview of general trends in English-language comics scholarship since the 1980s. This thumbnail sketch is not comprehensive, but instead aims to chart a number of important developments and turns in academic writing on comics.[5] One preliminary point is that much pioneering criticism was written not by academics, but by journalists, practitioners, fans, and enthusiasts. In the long view, the academy came late to comics studies. Since it has been taken up by academics, comics scholarship has generally followed familiar paths of development and traditional models of academic criticism in terms of its content and interests. Early studies from the 1970s and 1980s often worked to combat stubborn discrimination as they endeavored to establish the comics medium as a coherent and viable field of academic interest. Earlier publications were often quite specific in focus (such as Jules Feiffer's *The Great Comic Book Heroes*) or primarily archival (such as *The Smithsonian Collection of Newspaper Comics* and *A Smithsonian Book of Comic-Book Comics*).[6] These were important books, to be sure, especially as they presented older comics to new readers in a way that recognized and valued the history of the medium, but they were not what we would today typically recognize as scholarship or criticism.[7]

A number of more ambitious studies later moved beyond these more specialized predecessors: David Kunzle's monumental histories of comic strips, an ambitious survey of the early history of the English-language "picture story," beginning from the early days of print in the fifteenth century and continuing through the nineteenth century (in two volumes, 1973 and 1990); Martin Barker's *A Haunt of Fears*, which analyzed the ideological forces driving the 1950s British campaign against American crime and horror comics; and Joseph Witek's groundbreaking *Comic Books as History*, in which his formal readings of comics texts brought welcome critical rigor and insight.[8] As a representative group, these books exemplify a set of disciplinary approaches that have remained active in comics studies to the present day: historical and archival scholarship that charts a long prehistory and history for the medium; a cultural studies approach that considers how comics acquire significance through social use and exchange; and literary interpretation that balances formal analysis with a consideration of the medium as an ongoing and self-aware tradition. These books also show the great potential of interdisciplinary work in comics studies; such approaches can acknowledge and value the unique history and form of the medium in productive ways. And concurrent with these pioneering academic works, *The Comics Journal*, edited by Gary Groth, has long offered a lively forum—first in print and then online—for insightful coverage of comics. At its advent in the 1970s, *The Comics Journal* provided an important popular venue where writers, creators, and readers could discuss comics in an engaged and critical way.[9] By the end of the 1980s, serious criticism of comics had become a visible and viable enterprise.

Comics were suddenly on the academic map. More scholarly work appeared in the 1990s, some of it no doubt in response to the occasionally hyperbolic coverage of the emergence of the "graphic novel" as a sign that comics had achieved a transformative maturation, especially as evidenced by the publication of three titles in 1986–87: Frank Miller's *The Dark Knight Returns*, Alan Moore and David Gibbons's *Watchmen*, and the first volume of Art Spiegelman's *Maus* (each of which had appeared in serialized format prior to being published in book form). "Graphic novel," apparently coined in the 1960s, seems to have entered regular circulation as a marketing term in the 1970s, when it appeared on long-form comics like Richard Corben and Robert E. Howard's *Bloodstar*, but since then it has become an increasingly common descriptor for comics in general, most often with the misleading implication that the graphic novel represents a new kind of medium altogether.[10] The idea seems to have been that comics had finally evolved into a higher art form, one fitting for older, more serious readers. This often-repeated but reductive account of a sudden ascendancy—which designates a decisive historical turn coupled with the cachet of a new label—has proven quite resilient in both popular and academic writing on comics.

In 1993, Roger Sabin voiced an early criticism of this manufactured narrative in his *Adult Comics: An Introduction*, arguing that "the idea of an evolution from 'comics' to 'graphic novels' had a specific purpose—to add prestige to the form and thus to sell more product."[11] Moreover, Sabin contended that "for such a story to have had any currency, there had to be one crucial extra element—public ignorance . . . the general public has traditionally been profoundly unaware of the potential range of the comics medium, and has continued to see it essentially as entertainment for children."[12] Sabin mounts a useful critique of prepackaged narratives—such as the triumphal rise of the "graphic novel"—that are convenient and accessible but that ultimately misrepresent both comics and their history, often while masking the power of market forces. Despite its potentially misleading title, *Adult Comics* provided an important early intervention in comics criticism. The book offered a useful overview of the medium that aimed both to expand general knowledge and to challenge assumptions new and old. The general awareness of comics is undoubtedly much different today than it was in the early 1990s, but Sabin's hard-nosed criticism still encourages us to maintain a healthy skepticism of fossilized truisms about comics.

Also in 1993, cartoonist Scott McCloud published *Understanding Comics: The Invisible Art*, which remains perhaps the most widely read and cited book on comics to date.[13] McCloud's book, which is itself in the form of a comic, became something of a rallying point for comics studies. Like Kunzle and Sabin, McCloud proposes a long history of comics, which for him goes all the way back to cave paintings.[14] Building on Will Eisner's *Comics and Sequential Art*, McCloud offers an accessible vocabulary for analyzing comics as a visual medium with its own unique modes of signification.[15] *Understanding Comics* importantly draws attention to the formal aspects and visual grammar of comics, offering useful definitions, categories, and rubrics for thinking about comics in a more systematic and precise way. McCloud's book opened new possibilities for the study of comics: it asked readers to think about comics as a flexible and storied art form, and it offered a vocabulary for analyzing comics formally, one that has been readily adopted by many critics.[16]

Other notable publications from the 1990s include a number of essay collections by individual authors. M. Thomas Inge's *Comics as Culture* gathers a number of essays on comics (many of them previously published) that cover a range of topics and creators, including Winsor McCay, Krazy Kat, Charles Schulz, and EC science-fiction comics, along with a generous (and, for its time, comprehensive) annotated bibliography.[17] In his introduction, Inge makes a case for comics as "another form of legitimate culture" (xxi) but also underscores some of the difficulties facing comics criticism at the time: "This is the most difficult area to write about because we lack the critical vocabulary and have only begun to define the structural and stylistic principles behind successful comic art. Instead we tend to rely on terms borrowed from other areas of creative expression" (xviii). This particular challenge still occupies comics studies today. How can the field draw productively from other disciplines and critical vocabularies without losing a sense of its own particularity? How can comics studies both inform and be informed by other areas of intellectual and social interest?

Other significant essay collections from the 1990s include those of Robert C. Harvey (himself a cartoonist and a frequent contributor to *The Comics Journal*), *The Art of the Funnies* and *The Art of the Comic Book*. Both books outline and model ways of evaluating visual elements in comics with attention to what Harvey calls "visual-verbal blending." Harvey, like McCloud, broadcasts a bright sense of optimism and excitement for the future of comics, anticipating a "golden age" that lay "just ahead."[18] This was criticism charged with enthusiasm.

All the books from the 1990s surveyed above share certain features and interests: they offer some manner of historical overview for comics; they extend an introduction and invitation to comics; many of them include some theoretical content; and they work to justify comics as a "respectable" art form. All of these writers set out to educate a general audience about the comics medium—its history, its accomplishments, and its possibilities. In this sense, their writing functions as both criticism and advocacy. And while Inge has worked as an English professor, both McCloud and Harvey are writers and cartoonists, while Sabin was a journalist when he was invited to write *Adult Comics*.[19] A significant amount of this emergent scholarship on comics, then, was written not by academics but by practitioners and enthusiasts whose considerable learning and experience laid crucial groundwork, both historical and theoretical, for the continuing formation and development of comics studies. This diversity of backgrounds, vocations, and interests—and the range of expertise and the discourses that came along with it—made it possible for comics studies to move forward in productive ways.

The rising quality and quantity of comics scholarship in the 1980s and 1990s increased the status of the medium within the academic world. Whereas a good deal of the early scholarship had appeared under the rubric of cultural studies or popular culture, more and more scholars in other disciplines began to "do comics" in their work.[20] Indeed, beginning in the late 1990s and rapidly accelerating throughout the 2000s, something of a frontier spirit manifested as academic writers and publishers realized that a vast territory lay open before them, ready to be explored (and exploited) by enterprising spirits. Not surprisingly, some scholars, unwittingly or not, introduced careless errors and/or imported inherited attitudes about the "low" cultural value of comics as they moved to appropriate the newly available medium. Consider the following statement from Victoria Nelson, for example, which appears in her award-winning *The Secret Life of Puppets* (published in 2001 by Harvard University Press), wherein she considers the enduring presence of the spiritual and supernatural in popular media and entertainments: "In the 1980s comic books began to be translated from children's reading and matinee serial fare to the medium of adult mass movies. Comic books themselves had always attracted a shifting adult readership—from the crude pornography of the earliest forms though the counterculture comics of the 1960s to the sophisticated 'graphic novels' of the 1980s, such as *The Nightwatchman*, written by Alan Moore and drawn by Dave Gibbons, which feature an exaggerated cinematic style."[21] These sentences appear during a discussion of the migration of the supernatural from high to low culture in the United States during the twentieth century, part of a process that Nelson calls "the ghettoization of the American fantastic."[22] The most howling error here, of course, is the botched title for Moore and Gibbons's *Watchmen*, but the passage also recycles a worrying number of crusty assumptions and associations about comics in general: the development of "mature" comics, for example, begins with "crude pornography" (?) and ends with the "sophistication" of the "graphic novel" in the 1980s; the comparison between comics and film as a vague mode of praise for artistic accomplishment in the comics medium; and the seemingly indestructible idea that comics have evolved in fits and starts from children's fare to attract, finally, a "shifting" readership among adults. Indeed, the above passage presents a miniature case study of uninformed academic writing on comics. As we can see, the increased availability of comics to academic scholarship can yield unfortunate consequences when that scholarship is careless. While such egregious missteps are generally rare, it is still not uncommon to encounter errors that have escaped the vetting process of peer review and editing. By the end of the 1990s, many academics had become interested in comics, but not all of them possessed the expertise and diligence necessary to create scholarship of lasting value.

The 2000s then ushered in a flood of titles on comics from both popular and academic presses—guides, anthologies, readers, textbooks, reprints, and more.[23] Aimed at various audiences (fans, new and prospective readers, librarians, teachers, and scholars), the sheer number of such titles testifies to the explosive interest in comics in recent years. It is also noteworthy that both the National Council of Teachers of English (NCTE) and the Modern Language Association of America (MLA) have issued books to meet this burgeoning interest among their respective professional constituencies. Still, this mass of texts has generally remained dedicated to introducing comics to new readerships, to creating a corpus of notable content and creators, and to establishing comics as a legitimate area of intellectual interest. This current state of affairs indicates that comics studies is still very much occupied with announcing itself to the general public and defining (and justifying) itself as an academic field.

Within this prolonged start-up period, academic books dedicated to comics have tended to align themselves with established specializations and fields. This subscription to familiar paradigms has allowed easy recognition and dissemination across established disciplines, but it has also meant that the academic study of comics has largely been articulated through older critical movements and discourses.[24]

A number of scholars have been critical of this reflex. Bart Beaty, for example, has argued that "Comics Studies has so far failed to develop analytic and theoretical innovations that could be exported to cognate fields. Rather, it continues to rely on terminologies and theories handed down from other disciplines."[25] This is certainly not to devalue wholesale such a diverse body of scholarship, much of which has proven productive and insightful, but rather to underscore the point that recent scholarship has primarily articulated comics studies within or through already recognized systems of academic writing. Beginning in the late 1990s, many books on comics began to fall in line with established and comfortably familiar (at least to academics) fields in order to achieve quick legitimacy.

While the earlier work from the 1970s through the 1990s had established the groundwork for later scholarship, it had also tended to imagine a tradition marked by designations of periodization, generic categories and hierarchies, and major creators. This work of classification and definition formed a lasting catalogue of touchstones, transformations, and turning points that continues to define comics for academic consumption and use. Such a process clearly resembles traditional disciplinary formation. Comics scholarship, for example, has assembled a short list of master texts (think *Maus*, *Persepolis*, and *Fun Home*) and creators (think Will Eisner, R. Crumb, and Chris Ware) that constitutes a makeshift canon, despite the fact that the very notion of canonicity has fallen under scrutiny over the last several decades in literary studies. Canon formation traditionally favors certain genres and creators at the expense of others, an exclusionary process that risks producing an encoded elitism that can obscure or deny the multiplicity of comics.[26] In terms of genre, for example, memoir and nonfiction have been especially favored in recent academic studies of "literary" comics. This valuation has provoked some important debate over the status of particular genres in comics scholarship and the implications of generic privileging for the field.[27] Debates like these, which are essentially contests over appropriate content and direction, are indicative of a young field that remains preoccupied with marketing itself as a worthy subject of serious scholarship.

Comics as Serious/Literature/Art

This preoccupation with self-presentation and justification emerges in a number of ways, some of which I want to consider here. These areas include debates over terminology and classification (definition), rehearsals of the marginal status and/or the justification of comics (apology), and exaggeration of the medium's "potential" or "power" as culture, be it high or low or somewhere between (promotion). These reflexes must be at the very least interrogated, if not discarded, if comics studies is to move forward and produce enduring and far-ranging work. These preoccupations run the risk of overextending the field's preliminary moment, but—perhaps even more important—they can also keep scholars from reading and discussing actual comics (or even encourage them to continue circling the same insular group of established "worthy" texts). Tactics of generalization and/or celebration too often misrepresent comics and in the process limit the conversations we can have about the medium and its cultural significance. Through a focus on the general, we lose a sense of the particular and the possible.

The very fact that so little agreement exists on what to even call the medium testifies to the current self-consciousness in comics studies. Is the preferred term "graphic novel," "sequential art," "comics," "graphic lit," or "graphic narrative"? Many of these labels represent name-brand bids at a quick respectability that can somehow magically shed old stigmas and misconceptions. I prefer "comics" as a generally inclusive term that recognizes the medium's long history as a diverse popular form. Increasingly, however, academic writing has favored "graphic novel" over "comics," no doubt in part because the newer label implies a transformation from low to high culture. Despite its enduring use, however, "graphic novel" remains a notoriously imprecise descriptor. Artist and writer Eddie Campbell has nicely described the term as being

> currently used in at least four different and mutually exclusive ways. First, it is used simply as a synonym for comics books. . . . Second, it is used to classify a format—for example, a bound book of comics either in soft- or hardcover—in contrast to the old-fashioned stapled comic magazine. Third, it means, more specifically, a comic-book narrative that is equivalent in form and dimensions to the prose novel. Finally, others employ it to indicate a form that is more than a comic book in the scope of its ambition—indeed, a new medium altogether. It may be added that most of the important "graphic novelists" refuse to use the term under any conditions.[28]

Campbell sardonically outlines the problematic aspects of the term and its inconsistencies as a general catchall for comics in all their diversity of production, format, and content. Catherine Labio is likewise troubled by the term's ability to exclude certain work, arguing, "the eagerness with which the phrase 'graphic novel' has been adopted in academic writing points to a stubborn refusal to accept popular works on their own terms. 'Comics' reminds us of this vital dimension. 'Graphic novel' sanitizes comics; strengthens the distinction between high and low, major and minor; and reinforces the ongoing ghettoization of works deemed unworthy of critical attention, either because of their inherent nature . . . or because of their intended audience."[29] One problem with "graphic novel" as an inclusive term, then, is that it shuts out some forms of the medium: single issues and pamphlets, instructional comics, propaganda, web comics, minicomics, and so on. This omission both misrepresents the medium—its various forms, uses, and means of distribution—and devalues (intentionally or not) a broad range of material which does not neatly fit into predetermined models and expectations, many of which have been generated and sustained by fields and interests outside of comics.

Similar to the question of naming the medium—and sharing many of the same intellectual desires and evasions—is the debate over a proper definition for comics. Equally important to these enterprises is determining what the medium both can and cannot be. What counts as comics, and—perhaps more important—what is at stake in answering such a question? Working toward a definition of comics has proven both a productive and limiting exercise.[30] This dialogue has, if anything, increasingly suggested that while no definition of comics will ever prove satisfactory, each new one proposed advances its own restrictive set of value judgments. The question of definition has been with us at least since Coulton Waugh's early attempt in 1947, with its focus on comics as a form of mass entertainment, while the definition game has come under increasing scrutiny in recent years, especially since McCloud proposed his own definition in *Understanding Comics*.[31] McCloud influentially defined comics in this way: "Juxtaposed pictorial and other images in deliberate sequence, intended to convey information and/or to produce an aesthetic response in the viewer."[32] This versatile formulation avoids limiting aesthetic or value judgments, and it even encourages us to look for comics in places we might not expect to find them (although its insistence on sequence does preclude one-panel or single-image cartoons).

At the same time, McCloud's definition and methods have generated a good deal of debate, especially his committed effort to "separate form and content."[33] Cartoonist Dylan Horrocks, for example, has argued that McCloud "constructs a way of talking about comics that affirms and supports our longing for critical respectability and seems to offer an escape from the cultural ghetto."[34] This recuperative work occurs in part through an ambitious revision of the history of comics that distances popular and conventional genres from the "essential" form of the medium.[35] McCloud's definition "is more than simply a descriptive model," Horrocks argues; "it is also necessarily prescriptive. By reinforcing some values and suppressing others, it can influence the way we read and create comics, discouraging experimentation in some directions and imposing particular narrative structures and idioms."[36] Horrocks writes as a cartoonist, and his concerns consequently turn on the creative choices and possibilities for making comics, but his reservations are relevant, as well, to the work of criticism and its potential avenues of investigation and circulation.

The prescriptive element of definition appears frequently in academic writing on comics. Hillary Chute, for example, in an essay published in *PMLA* (the flagship journal for literary studies), defines comics as "a hybrid word-and-image form in which two narrative tracks, one verbal and one visual, register temporality spatially."[37] Chute's succinct definition, couched in academic discourse, notably imagines the medium's form as separate from its history.[38] Her definition—along with her use of "graphic narrative" as a preferred term for nonfiction comics, in her opinion "the strongest genre in the field"—seems specifically designed to appeal to the academic readers of *PMLA*; at the same time, however, much as McCloud does in his own way, Chute implicitly separates the medium from its popular past and thus presents it as serious fare for serious scholarship. Moreover, through the work of discourse and the strategic selection of texts, Chute transmutes comics (or at least nonfiction comics) into "literature."

Indeed, the "comics as literature" credo became increasingly prominent (if not clichéd) throughout the 2000s.[39] In *This Book Contains Graphic Language: Comics as Literature*, for example, Rocco Versaci argues that comics represent "a sophisticated literary art form," formulating his position through a series of comparisons between comics and other genres and media, such as memoir, photography, film, and literature.[40] As one reviewer has noted, this comparative approach "is intended to loan comics some of the legitimacy of the established work, but the implicit suggestion is that comics are only worthy of serious consideration *because* they resemble the accepted literature."[41] In other words, comics gain value only through their association with other art forms—they are defined and discussed through the properties of other media rather than as their own particular form. Such a model of interpretation runs the risk of passing over aspects and potentials that are unique or especially well suited to the medium of comics. Why must comics be coded as "literature"? Leaving aside difficult questions of how even to define literature, the motive behind naming comics in this way is clear enough: to acquire a transformative legitimacy through a change of nomenclature. Moreover, naming comics as literature suggests that scholars can easily and without distortion apply existing discourses of literary criticism to comics.[42]

But what do such shortcuts mean for our understanding and appreciation of the medium? What might we lose when comics become literature? In part, the championing of comics as literature imports hoary standards of aesthetic excellence, genius, and innovation. It can also promote the valuation of certain genres and creators at the expense of others. Calling comics "literature" begs an immediate credibility, but it does not accomplish the real work of thinking about comics as an artistic medium with its own history, forms of signification, and cultural uses.

These strategic definitions and name games all emerge in part from the uneasy awareness that comics were not considered a high art form in the United States for most of the twentieth century. Comics, we are incessantly reminded, were, for a long while, disposable entertainments, the trashy heirs of pulp magazines, written for the masses and churned out for profit. Scholars have worked very hard to dispel this negative association even as they repeatedly call attention to its existence. In the opening sentence of her *PMLA* essay, for example, Chute writes, "Comics—a form once considered pure junk—is sparking interest in literary studies."[43] The implication seems to be that comics have finally moved away from the vulgar and into the literary. New art forms, of course, have always inspired suspicion or been measured against, or (de)valued through, already established forms, models, and paradigms. Consider, for example, the low opinion of the novel that was common in the eighteenth century, as evidenced in the comments of Thomas Jefferson in a letter written in March 1818:

> A great obstacle to good education is the inordinate passion prevalent for novels, and the time lost in that reading which should be instructively employed. When this poison infects the mind, it destroys its tone and revolts it against wholesome reading. Reason and fact, plain and unadorned, are rejected. Nothing can engage attention unless dressed in all the figments of fancy, and nothing so bedecked comes amiss. The result is a bloated imagination, sickly judgment, and disgust towards all the real businesses of life. This mass of trash, however, is not without some distinction; some few modelling their narratives, although fictitious, on the incidents of real life, have been able to make them interesting and useful vehicles of a sound morality.[44]

Such attitudes might strike us today as anachronistic, but Jefferson's distinction between "trash" and "useful" reading is familiar enough. In many ways, Jefferson's outlook recalls the recent privileging of graphic memoir and nonfiction works in academic writing on comics. Such texts, perhaps because they are not "fanciful," can be taken seriously. One can read Spiegelman, Satrapi, and Bechdel without embarrassment, the idea goes, because they transcend the "mass of trash" by virtue of being part of a new comics literature that draws from "the incidents of real life." Classifying comics as literature—or celebrating a particular work, genre, or creator—can be the valid work of criticism, but when these reflexes proceed from insecurities over the cultural position of comics, they run the risk of prolonging or perpetuating many of the obstacles that comics studies has worked to overcome, especially when scholarship marginalizes parts of the medium in order to justify what it considers to be serious or literary—or art.

Finally, the imperative to establish comics as literature has led many well-intentioned scholars to celebrate the medium in exaggerated terms. Such boosterism can be self-defeating. Consider the example of Stephen E. Tabachnick's essay "A Comic-Book World," which proposes several reasons why the graphic novel stands uniquely poised to eclipse, slowly but surely, the reading of books without pictures. The essay contains a number of dubious claims, such as its statement that *Watchmen* is "known as the *Ulysses* of the graphic novel for its subtlety, stylistic variety, philosophical reach, and depth of characterization, and which is much more approachable than Joyce's *Ulysses*," and later, that Moore and Gibbons "prove that verbal and visual poets can indeed be seers, as the Romans believed."[45] Such reckless overstatement stands little chance of winning the lasting interest of skeptics (or even the casually interested). And what does it mean that all the images in Tabachnick's essay come from recent film adaptations of comics texts? The essay primarily (and problematically) discusses comics through something else—film, video games, 9/11, traditional literature, electronic reading, and so on. Indeed, we never see any actual comics in the essay. Overselling the medium in this way, without ever representing comics themselves, relies too much on often-repeated and easily anticipated talking points rather than on responsible and convincing analysis. For comics studies to move forward, we must stop appropriating value for comics through associations with other media and art forms. We need not valorize comics at the expense of rhetorical credibility.

The recurrent problems and pitfalls in comics criticism that I survey here generally proceed from the lingering perception that scholars must justify comics to an assumed audience of doubters and naysayers. These defensive reflexes, I contend, are both unnecessary and counterproductive. Academics are trained to think within established critical disciplines and to write primarily for other academics within those disciplines. One of the most exciting aspects of comics studies, however, is its potential to speak both to and beyond any one audience. As we have seen, comics criticism began in the public domain, and it still thrives there today. Aaron Meskin has called attention to the high quality of comics coverage in magazines and newspapers, for example, which can often "amount to more than reports of preferences. This is fully fledged criticism—albeit in compact form."[46] Likewise, a wealth of critical insight and expertise appears daily on online blogs and forums.[47] And finally, as Greg Smith has observed of comics scholarship in general, "Some of the most useful published work comes from those who are outside of the academy because as writer-artists, they pay close attention to the production, distribution, and circulation contexts."[48] University scholars have much to learn about comics from nonacademic writers and practitioners.

Comics studies has the potential to speak to a heterogeneous audience with various interests and backgrounds. Consider, for example, the mission statement of the Institute for Comics Studies, which works "to promote the study, understanding, recognition, and cultural legitimacy of comics through communications within the scholarly, professional, and fan communities, and with the general public."[49] The Sequart Research and Literacy Organization likewise describes itself as a group that "publishes scholarly non-fiction books on subjects related to the medium of sequential art. Our books attempt to be scholarly but accessible to a general audience. We specialize in literary analysis that avoids the insularity that can typify academic writing, trying instead to open critical discourse on comics to a wider, intelligent audience."[50] Initiatives like these imagine a middle voice capable of speaking to multiple audiences. They also suggest that comics scholarship need not always follow well-blazed byways in order to navigate a short path to respectability. We need not transform comics into "literature" through the alchemy of discourse. Instead, we might look at comics more on their own terms even as we consider the different ways in which people read, create, distribute, and value comics. And, although it should go without saying, we must simply read more comics (certainly more than *Maus*, *Persepolis*, and *Fun Home*). We might think about how comics work formally, yes, but also how they are made and experienced by different communities of creators and consumers and how they acquire value through use and circulation.[51] Since comics are a popular art born from a mass medium, shouldn't comics studies also be pluralist in its interests and methodologies, considering how comics work as social objects that are used, exchanged, and/or contested by different groups?

Such a model of criticism can aspire to analysis that includes but thinks beyond comics as textual artifacts or as art objects that invite and reward interpretation, in order to consider also a multiplicity of uses, communities, business models, and institutional forces as well as influences and intersections outside of comics.[52] This method might more freely include comics that do not conveniently demonstrate well-established attributes of the literary (e.g., memoir, "serious" matter, artistic excellence, formal innovation) as well as comics that come from multiple forms of distribution and consumption (online comics, strips, minicomics, small print runs, periodicals or floppies, personal work or work intended for limited circulation, and so on). From my own perspective as a literature scholar, this might mean attention to the ethical and social functions as well as to the aesthetic aspects of comics. Rather than championing canonical texts and creators, privileging certain kinds of narratives (especially those that fit comfortably within learned expectations of the literary), or even attending primarily to formal innovation, we might ask how comics work among and for a diverse public readership.

In closing, this essay calls for an open discourse that values collaboration over competition, inclusion over exclusion. By considering comics as cultural objects situated within and across different networks (social, institutional, textual, experiential, and so on), we can begin to answer Joseph Witek's longstanding call for "critical discourse to use the conceptual tools at hand to examine the connections between the specific textual attributes of comics and the social, economic, and ideological matrices in which they are enmeshed."[53] Such a broad vision would effectively interrogate the cultural formation and value of the literary—and the place of comics within that ambiguous field—and consequently reengage literature with the social realm. The time has come for comics criticism to reflect the range, energy, and innovation of its subject.

· · · · · · · ·

Nate Powell's *Swallow Me Whole* offers one example of a long-form comic that represents the variable experience of illness in several characters and raises questions over how standard medical discourse and diagnosis might be incomplete in response to those experiences. We especially see this effect when the character Ruth is diagnosed as schizophrenic by her doctor, who most often looks down at a desk when explaining the condition, its diagnosis, and the debate currently surrounding the "disorder." Interspersed throughout the scene are silent images of Ruth's brother, Perry, as he is elsewhere assaulted by another teenager and then interrogated by a passing police officer. Side-by-side panels show a simultaneous moment as Ruth receives a prescription from her doctor (the form is covered in illegible scribbles) and Perry reads a written citation from the policeman. This visual joining suggests an uncertainty in the diagnosis and treatment of mental illness, with additional associations of violence and institutional failure arising through the juxtaposition of the two scenes on the page.

Partial representation and silences in each scenario also mean that the reader must extrapolate from fragmentary evidence in order to assign meaning to the sequence. The side-by-side juxtaposition of prescription (physician) and citation (police officer) combines intimations of treatment, punishment, judgment, shame, and guilt, all of which are determined by the authority that diagnoses a situation or condition and then issues an official response in writing. This compelling scene calls attention to the multiple aspects and positions that shape the interpretation of texts, persons, and conditions. And when the penultimate panel assumes Ruth's perspective as she receives her inscrutable prescription, the comic deftly challenges the reader to make sense of the text that he or she has been given. These pages accordingly invite the reader to both interpretation and empathy.

FIGURES ON
FOLLOWING PAGES

▬ ▬ ▬ ▬ ▬ ▬

figs. 1.1–1.4
From Nate Powell, *Swallow Me Whole*
(Marietta, GA: Top Shelf, 2008).

fig. 1.1

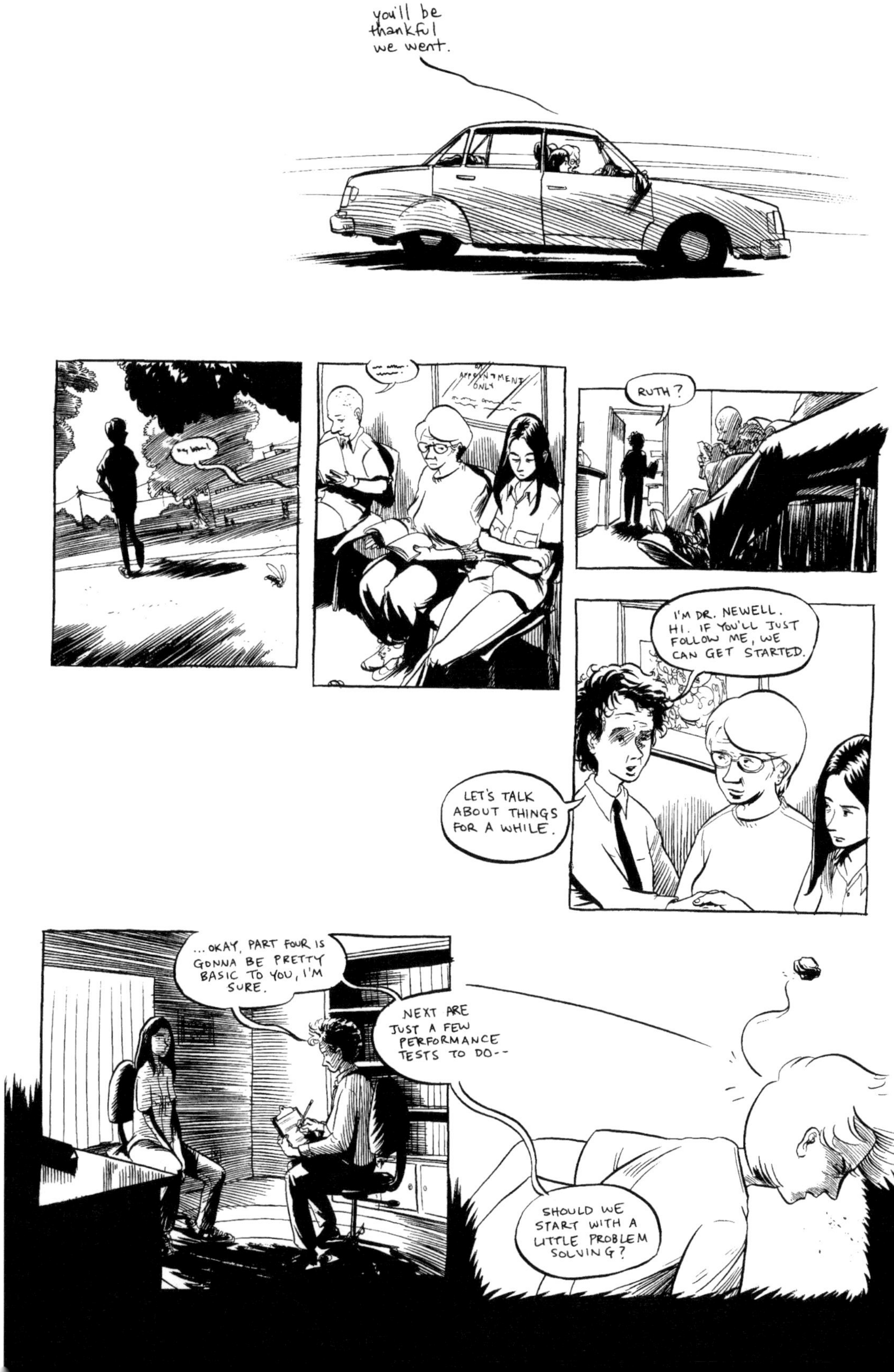
you'll be thankful we went.
RUTH?
I'M DR. NEWELL. HI. IF YOU'LL JUST FOLLOW ME, WE CAN GET STARTED.
LET'S TALK ABOUT THINGS FOR A WHILE.
...OKAY, PART FOUR IS GONNA BE PRETTY BASIC TO YOU, I'M SURE.
NEXT ARE JUST A FEW PERFORMANCE TESTS TO DO--
SHOULD WE START WITH A LITTLE PROBLEM SOLVING?

fig. 1.2

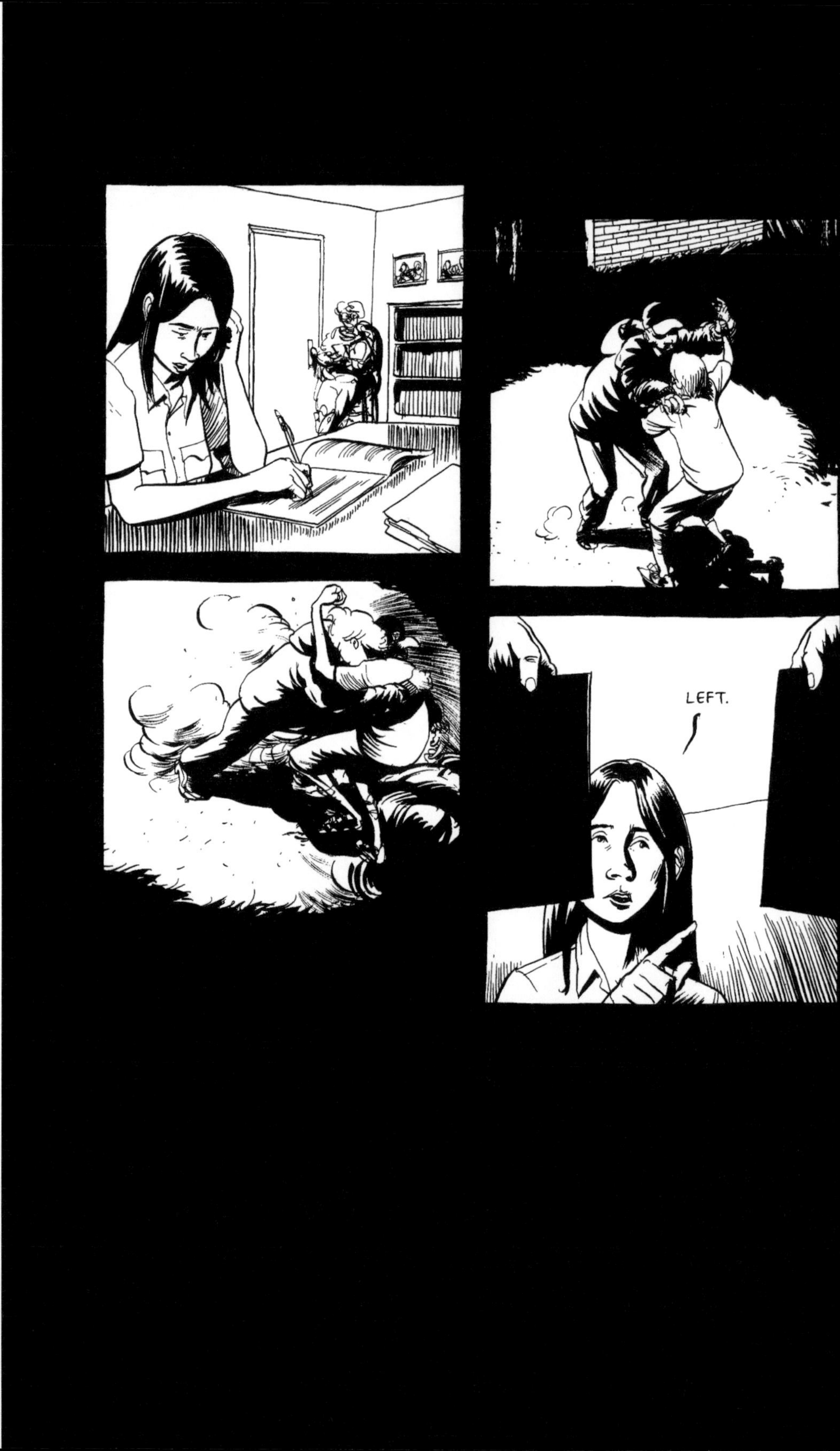
LEFT.

fig. 1.3

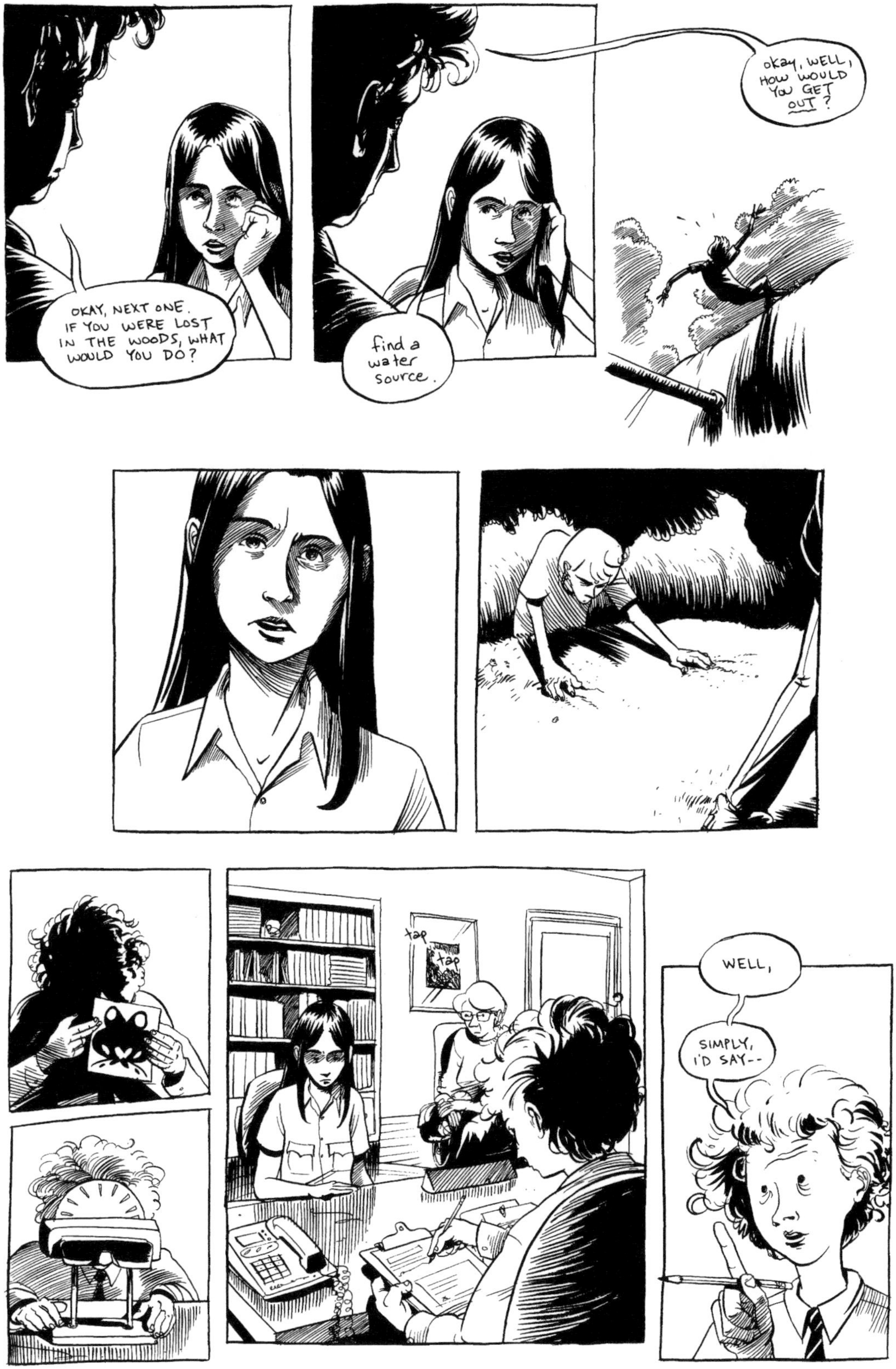
OKAY, NEXT ONE. IF YOU WERE LOST IN THE WOODS, WHAT WOULD YOU DO?
find a water source.
okay, WELL, HOW WOULD YOU GET OUT?
tap
tap
WELL,
SIMPLY, I'D SAY--

who gets to speak?

fig. 1.4

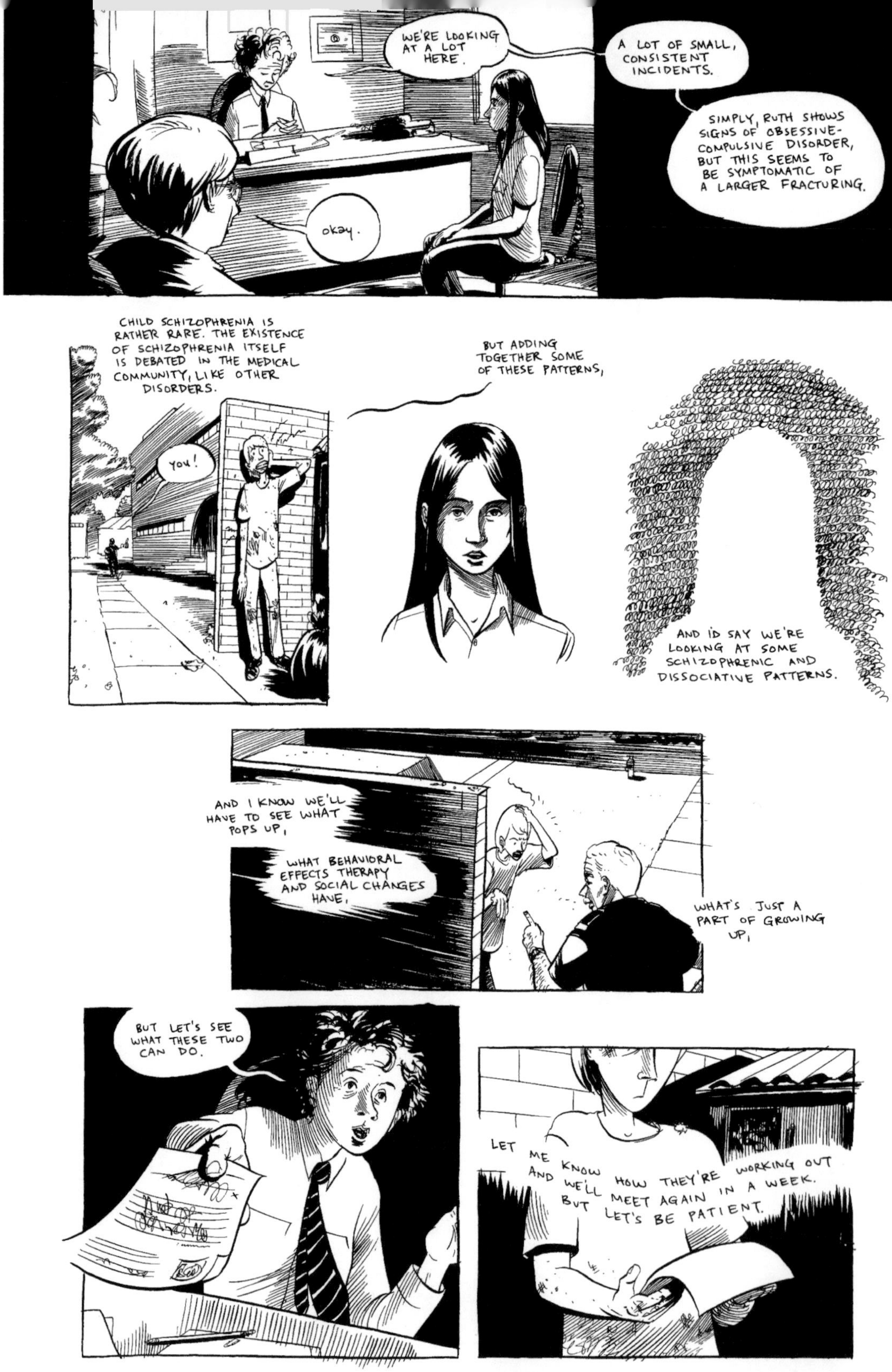
WE'RE LOOKING AT A LOT HERE.
A LOT OF SMALL, CONSISTENT INCIDENTS.
SIMPLY, RUTH SHOWS SIGNS OF OBSESSIVE-COMPULSIVE DISORDER, BUT THIS SEEMS TO BE SYMPTOMATIC OF A LARGER FRACTURING.
okay.
CHILD SCHIZOPHRENIA IS RATHER RARE. THE EXISTENCE OF SCHIZOPHRENIA ITSELF IS DEBATED IN THE MEDICAL COMMUNITY, LIKE OTHER DISORDERS.
YOU!
BUT ADDING TOGETHER SOME OF THESE PATTERNS,
AND I'D SAY WE'RE LOOKING AT SOME SCHIZOPHRENIC AND DISSOCIATIVE PATTERNS.
AND I KNOW WE'LL HAVE TO SEE WHAT POPS UP,
WHAT BEHAVIORAL EFFECTS THERAPY AND SOCIAL CHANGES HAVE,
WHAT'S JUST A PART OF GROWING UP,
BUT LET'S SEE WHAT THESE TWO CAN DO.
LET ME KNOW HOW THEY'RE WORKING OUT AND WE'LL MEET AGAIN IN A WEEK. BUT LET'S BE PATIENT.

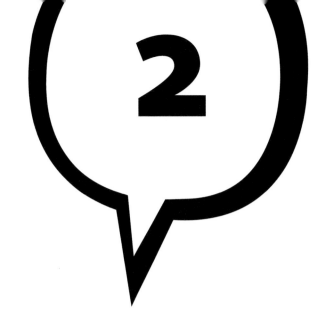

The Uses of Graphic Medicine for Engaged Scholarship

Susan Merrill
Squier

Comics were an illicit pleasure for me when I was a girl. In my house, reading was restricted to "literature," but my neighbors—Lindy, who was my age, and Sandy, her older sister—had stacks of comics in the bedroom they shared. When I spent the night at their house, I would sit on the floor under the glassy-eyed surveillance of their Ginny dolls and read comic after comic—*Archie, Betty and Veronica, Little Lulu*, and occasionally *Superman* or *Batman*.[1] In those comics-reading splurges that were never long enough, I would muse over the mysteries of teenage life— would Archie end up with blonde Betty or sultry dark-haired Veronica? Where would I fit into that world, as neither a Betty nor a Veronica? Why—when he seemed so much more interesting than Archie—wasn't Jughead also in the running for a girlfriend? The mysteries of gender and sexuality seemed just out of reach in Bob Montana's cheerfully Comics Code–compliant series.

When I was in my early teens, my younger brother brought home Kurtzman's *MAD* magazine and I was hooked for years. Later, discovering *Mr. Natural* as a college student in 1968 felt like stumbling through a familiar door that opened on a new source of illicit pleasure—to go right along with marijuana and sex.[2] In those years, I read comics that fed my growing commitment to social justice issues: the draft, the war, and, finally, feminism. (I never came across a comic that addressed the civil rights movement.) But this was only in my free time. I was studying English literature by then—Shakespeare, Coleridge, Dickens, and Conrad—and I took it for granted that comics related to a different part of my brain and a different part of my life as well. True, I still bellied down with the Sunday funnies religiously, but other than that I didn't read comics for a long time.

Or so I like to think. Yet I remember that I have been a fan of *Doonesbury* from its very first strip in 1970, and I have a screen memory of reading *Dykes to Watch Out For* (*DTWOF*) right next to *Stan Mack's Real Life Funnies* and Jules Feiffer's strips in the *Village Voice* in the late 1970s.[3] But that must just be wishful thinking, since Alison Bechdel didn't publish the first *DTWOF* strip until 1983, and never in the *Village Voice*.

Comics continued as sotto-voce accompaniment to my graduate training as a Virginia Woolf scholar and a modernist. Although I wasn't reading many super-hero comics at this point—they had been gendered male since my Archie and Veronica 'fifties—I devoured *Doonesbury* (still do), *The Far Side*, and, later, *For Better or for Worse*.[4] Yet even after I discovered *Maus*, comics were still something I kept separate from my work life.[5] I was doing research in women's studies, science studies, and literature and medicine, areas that appealed to me because I could an-alyze literature and culture as a way into social, political, and environmental issues. Cartoonlike illustrations from the pulp science-fiction magazine *Amazing Stories* played a part in my 1994 book, *Babies in Bottles*. But I only began to incorporate comics in my scholarship when I stumbled upon two comics that brilliantly cap-tured how society and biomedical science together were reshaping the structure and significance of human life: Tom Tomorrow's "Immortality for Achievers" and Ruben Bolling's "Bad Blastocyst."[6]

The former captured the debate over organ transplantation in just six stinging panels. A G. W. Bush presidential initiative, "Immortality for Achievers," proposes the "harvesting [of] vital organs from the poor" in order to "prolong life for the wealthy." Although Congress and TV pundits both debate the proposal and "a few crazy extremists insist that both parties are somehow 'in thrall' to their 'wealthy contributors,'" a "bipartisan consensus is achieved" and the "Mandatory Organ Donation Act of 2002" is passed, under which "next of kin will receive a gift cer-tificate worth FIVE DOLLARS off their next purchase at ANY government surplus facility." A prescient final panel shows a perspiring Dick Cheney leaning in to the image and commanding, "Now somebody get me a new TICKER—and I mean PRONTO!"[7]

After including a discussion of "Immortality for Achievers" in my *Liminal Lives*, I returned to comics in the volume's coda with Bolling's "Bad Blastocyst," a pitch-perfect satire of the contemporary debate over stem-cell experimentation.[8] The comic introduces us to the case at "Sal's Fertility Clinic n' Stuff," in which a petri dish containing a blastocyst—a five- or six-day-old embryo—is acciden-tally knocked off a cabinet by a cleaning woman. It "falls on her head, killing her instantly. BONK!" The blastocyst is charged with murder, and the ensuing trial provokes media coverage that raises increasingly challenging (if designedly absurd) legal, social, and medical issues (*Liminal Lives*, 269). "Bad Blastocyst" can fuel an ethics seminar in just ten panels.

I had discovered the power of comics, although my awareness of literary hierarchies was also still present in that analysis of "Bad Blastocyst." In *Liminal Lives*, I categorized comics as "perhaps the most highly stigmatized fictional genre" before going on to assert that "this brief comic strip reveals how stem cells can be used to raise issues as diverse as the legal definition of a rights-bearing subject, the questions of psychological and social responsibility, and the rationale for, and goal of, scientific research" (268). Arguing then that the comics medium is so powerful because it enables us simultaneously to articulate and disavow risky, disturbing, or even taboo ideas, I implicitly accepted a view of comics that situated the medium as a zone beyond serious conversation.

Yet I learned how effective comics could be in communicating serious biomedical issues as I gave talks following the publication of *Liminal Lives*. Audiences relaxed, freed from the straitjacket of academic prose, and seemed to enjoy considering the conflicting forces in stem-cell research when they encountered them embodied in "Bad Blastocyst." Excited by the powerful mixture of pleasure and knowledge made possible by this yeasty medium that Ian Williams would later call "graphic medicine,"[9] I began to explore how comics could enhance "engaged scholarship," the dry shorthand for research that falls outside traditional departmental offerings. The concept was popularized by Ernest Boyer of the Carnegie Foundation for the Advancement of Teaching. In Boyer's 1990 report, *Scholarship Reconsidered: Priorities of the Professoriate*, he urged academics to strive for communication and even collaboration with the nonacademic public. With that exhortation, the activism already integral to social movements and the applied professions found an authorized route into the humanities and social sciences sectors of the university.

While graphic medicine may seem most closely tied to the medical humanities, a closer look will reveal its relevance to fields of engaged scholarship beyond the medical or health humanities. This category includes women's studies, environmental studies, disability studies, and science and technology studies, as well as critical race studies, queer studies, and animal studies. Each of these areas has a mandate for real-world commitment and engagement that comics can serve well. In what follows, I will give some examples of the kinds of challenging questions an alternative comics perspective has raised for several of these scholarly fields, and I'll also discuss the rich role comics can play there in teaching. But first, a quick word about how comics found their way into my own work in the medical humanities and went on to illuminate the health humanities.

engaged
scholarship

From the Medical to the Health Humanities

In July 1997, Kathryn Montgomery and Tod Chambers of the Medical Humanities and Bioethics Department at Northwestern University's Feinberg School of Medicine offered a weeklong seminar: Case History, Narrative, and the Construction of Objectivity. I participated in that bioethics seminar four weeks after I had undergone a hysterectomy-oophorectomy in response to an excruciating ovarian torsion. With my own recent surgical experience much on my mind, I was happy to encounter a cartoonist, the artist Ann Starr, among the remarkable scholar-practitioners participating in the seminar. In her powerful artist's book, "Where Babies Come From: A Miracle Explained," she explored the socially and medically charged experience of the hysterectomy in a way that spoke directly to my own still very confused feelings about my recent surgery. I was inspired by the vivid access to the medical experience that Starr's art exemplified, and I went on to collaborate with her on a hybrid-form essay and proto-comic, "Speaking Women's Bodies: A Conversation," which appeared the following year in *Literature and Medicine*.

Five years later, Anne Hunsaker Hawkins and I offered our own seminar, Medicine, Literature, and Culture, under the auspices of the National Endowment for the Humanities (NEH). Working in a borrowed office in the Humanities Department of the Penn State College of Medicine—just two doors down from a co-author of this volume, Michael Green (whom I had yet to meet)—I spent that month co-teaching a diverse group of college professors. They had joined us for four weeks of intensive classroom discussions and hours shadowing healthcare professionals at Hershey Medical Center (the Neonatal Intensive Care Unit, the Emergency Room, and the ICU), as well as weekly meditation sessions I led and play-reading gatherings Starr hosted. One of these professors was another co-author of this volume, Kimberly Myers.

During that extended immersion in the medical humanities, we were joined by other Hershey Medical Center colleagues—I well remember Michael Green's presentation on the ethics of the patient interview—as well as some outside visitors.[10] Among them were Rita Charon from the Columbia University Program in Narrative Medicine, Chambers and Montgomery from the Medical Humanities and Bioethics Department at Northwestern, and Starr. As she had five years earlier at the Northwestern seminar, Starr presented "Where Babies Come From" to our seminar group, offering an early glimpse of the power of comics in the medical or health humanities.

That NEH seminar had taken place under the auspices of the oldest medical humanities program in the United States, launched in 1967 when Joanne Trautmann Banks was appointed to the new Humanities Department at the Penn State College of Medicine. In its early years, work in the developing field of medical humanities often relied on history and philosophy to illuminate the practice of medicine. Anne Hunsaker Hawkins contributed the important concept of "pathography," a narrative of illness; Suzanne Poirier argued for the need to enrich the medical chart by drawing on the crucial role of nurses in patient care; and Kathryn Montgomery (Hunter) illuminated the epistemological foundations of medical diagnosis, pointing to the importance of narrative thinking, case-based storytelling, and a Sherlock Holmesian search for clues as the set of productive practices characterizing medical reasoning. As the medical humanities developed, it engendered narrative medicine. Locating its practice at the point of encounter between patient and healthcare practitioner, this new area of inquiry, more strongly grounded in literature, aimed at strengthening clinical practice by providing practitioners with the "narrative competence to recognize, absorb, metabolize, interpret, and be moved by the stories of illness."[11] Although the field styled itself as emerging organically "from individuals' ethics practices as they . . . found themselves listening in new ways to their patients and thinking in new ways about cases," it owes much to the pioneering influence of its founder, physician and literary scholar Rita Charon.[12] With its explicit address to the medical community, Charon's advocacy of narrative as a mode of thought that could improve medical reasoning made powerful headway into medical school curricula. Physicians and medical students together began to experiment with how to narrate—and thus illuminate—their experiences interacting with and treating their patients.

Recent scholarship has drawn attention to the visual as well as verbal representations of disease and health. As media studies scholar Kirsten Ostherr argues, the perspectives of narrative medicine and medical humanities must be blended if we are to "engage the full spectrum of discourses engaged in shaping our understandings of health and disease."[13] Noting that the relevance and scope of the field would be broadened by the incorporation of biocultural studies—a field of Foucault-inflected scholarship inaugurated by Lennard Davis and David Morris, whose interdisciplinary approach includes attention to visual representations of disease and health—Ostherr urges scholars in both narrative medicine and medical humanities to engage with phenomena ranging from anatomical illustrations, photographs, and medical visualization technologies (X-rays, ultrasounds, MRIs, PET scans, CT scans, fMRIs) to films (photographic and animated, educational and popular), videos, art exhibits, television programs, and social media.[14]

Ostherr surprisingly omits any mention of comics in her study *Medical Visions: Producing the Patient Through Film, Television, and Imaging Technologies*, although she includes animations among the visual representations that a biocultural approach to medicine might examine. Yet as students of animation know, the animated cartoon itself developed from the newspaper comic strip in the United States, so it would not be a stretch to equate the value of animation with that of comics. Indeed, animation scholars John Halas and Roger Manvell point out, in what might be misread as an explicit allusion to the pedagogical power of graphic medicine, that "where live action particularizes, animation generalizes, and in the process makes what it seeks to explain universal."[15] In the very terms of Ostherr's study, comics offer a powerful medium to bring biocultural analyses of medicine, as well as of health humanities, to a wide audience. Comics, with their unique treatment of time, enable precisely the kind of extralinguistic, visually based analysis Ostherr affirms as essential for a biocultural approach to experience.

Practitioners of narrative medicine are keenly aware of the force of time, which they understand as the medium of life itself. In a beautiful meditation called "Time and Ethics," Charon argues this point: "Human beings are held aloft in a time that 'flows,' unaware except at the bidding of illness or of art how beholden we are to the buoyancy of our medium; without its invisible hand, we sink like stones into death."[16] Practitioners encounter stories of illness richly saturated with temporality, whether it is the clinical time of case histories, the anxious or hopeful time of patient pathographies, or the reflective time of family or caregiver assessments. Arguing that both medicine and bioethics "must be captured in narrative in order to be beheld in their organic, timeful whole," Charon and Martha Montello describe the ethical agenda for narrative medicine: listen to the patient's story; attend to the expectations, wishes, and fears expressed; and try to enable the patient to shape a meaningful life, right up to its end.

Yet the context of narrative medicine shapes the concept of time in ways that are worth considering. The form of time that to Charon contains the most powerfully charged meaning is diachronic time, the perception of time as a flow within which the narrator experiences his or her embodied self. Significantly, Charon dismisses another form of time as irrelevant to the project of narrative medicine: synchronic time. Grouping together "the propositional thinking of moral philosophy, the epiphanic awareness of some forms of poetry, [and] the synchronic (that is to say, simultaneous or all-at-once) perception of the visual arts," Charon argues that they all depart from "the kind of human knowledge expressible through and experienced in narrative" (Charon and Montello, *Stories Matter*, 59). Her dismissal comes too quickly, however. Because the medium of comics represents time spatially, it offers the advantage of being able to incorporate the rich human knowledge experienced in synchronic time as well as the narrative access to diachronic time. Panels combining images and words can represent events synchronically even as the textual narrative of the comic is floating down the diachronic river. While narrative medicine focuses on the textual and verbal, graphic medicine can access those aspects of illness and medicine that we experience visually and spatially, as enduring, if intractable, aspects of the patient experience.

Consider, for example, how Brian Fies represents the imperative diagnostic touch of a uniquely medical interchange in *Mom's Cancer*.[17] Mom's neurological exam is presented on one page, in images arrayed synchronically to accompany

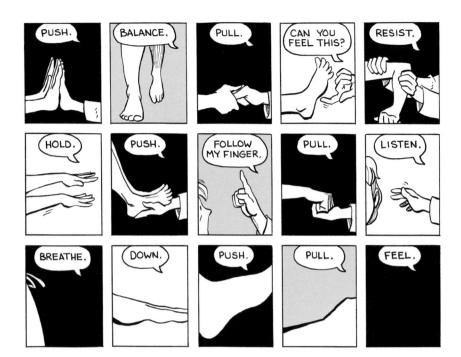

fig. 2.1
From Brian Fies, *Mom's Cancer* (New
York: Abrams Image, 2006).

the diachronic stream of verbal narrative, with the result that the reader's attention is drawn from diagnostic distance to empathy. Alternating black, white, and gray images—in three tiered rows of five panels each—present the sequential physical encounters of a neurological exam (fig. 2.1). Each panel contains the command, the relevant bit of Mom's body, and at times the physician's hands. The commands—"Push," "Balance," "Pull," "Can you feel this?" and "Resist"—are layered over others—"Hold," "Push," "Follow my finger," "Pull," and "Listen" (18). Sedimented at the bottom of these layers, we find another row of commands: "Breathe," "Down," "Push," "Pull," and finally, at the far right, "Feel" (18).

While comics conventions dictating the typical reading order of left-to-right and top-to-bottom incorporate the expected diachronic sequence, the representation of the examination on one page, able to be read all at once, introduces a synchronic rendering as well. Layering different modes of experience in complex interplay, the panels are simultaneously visible as well as sequentially experienced: "Push," "Pull," and "Listen" linger in the mind, to be moved through and also grasped at the same time as "Feel" (18). With that last command, the uncomfortable impingement, disjointed seriality, and effortful actions of Mom's encounter with her physician give way to a fully black panel where we see neither part of Mom's body nor her doctor's hands. Instead, as we read and internalize the action, the command "Feel" links us (as readers) to Mom (as patient) through its ironically resonant double meaning.

As this graphic example suggests, with the turn to the health humanities, the focus of the field has expanded from an implicit endorsement of the practitioner's emphasis on medical treatment to a critical incorporation of the caregiver's or patient's experiences, including the social determinants of health and well-being. Consider just three institutional markers of this change, all occurring within less than a decade. In 2006, two major conferences occurred that began what might be called a post-positivist shift in perspective on these issues: a think tank on Emergent Paradigms in Women's Health, hosted by the Women's College Research Institute at the University of Toronto and co-organized by neuroscientist Gillian Einstein and philosopher Margrit Shildrick, and a conference on the Health Humanities, hosted by Green College of the University of British Columbia and co-organized by English professor Judy Segal and philosopher Alan Richardson. In both gatherings, scholars drew on the historical and literary groundings of the medical humanities while introducing new perspectives and new sources in order to formulate what might be called a "critical health studies," attentive to gender-, race-, class-, and age-based power discrepancies. Such a health humanities–grounded approach attends not only to the intersectional factors shaping the relations between patient and caregiver but also to the power of unorthodox sources, including comics, to convey meanings otherwise overlooked in conventional medical humanities scholarship.

Just eight years later, in 2014, a two-day Obermann Working Symposium at the University of Iowa called Health Humanities: Building the Future in Research and Teaching convened several researchers and artists, asking them to assess the state of the field of health humanities and chart its future. The participants included the editors of two forthcoming anthologies of scholarship and creative work in the health humanities, an artist who inaugurated the use of art to deepen the visual and emotional awareness of medical students and doctors, a co-founder of a pathbreaking program in narrative medicine, a co-director of a noted center for literature and medicine, and a co-editor of a graphic medicine series.[18] The symposium addressed many issues, from educating smarter health consumers and more patient-focused clinicians, to increasing awareness of the experiential components of health and wellness, to enhancing what one participant called "practical compassion." "What are we bringing to the table, when we work in the Health Humanities?" the participants were asked. They pointed to inter- and multidisciplinary projects offering very different ways of being and acting specific to healthcare and well-being, incorporating joy, and drawing on the strategies of deep play. As this formulation suggests, whether we call it medical humanities, narrative medicine, biocultural studies, or the health humanities, the field now engages both the power of the visual and the force of knowledges and practices extending far beyond institutional medicine. In the rest of this chapter, I will suggest the role graphic medicine can play in some

graphic medicine
manifesto

48

of the most powerful inter- and multidisciplinary sites of work in the health humanities.

Disability Studies

At its core, disability studies (DS) is a mode of engaged scholarship and teaching. DS has traditionally distinguished between the medical and social models for explaining the origin and proper response to a disability. Viewed from a medical perspective, a disability may be either congenital or acquired, but it requires treatment by healthcare professionals until it has been ameliorated or cured. In contrast, the social model of disability holds that a person's impairment (whatever its etiology) becomes a disability only if and when the social environment fails to accommodate it. This extends from mores that stigmatize people with disabilities to built environments that restrict access by people with disabilities. Recently some DS scholars have argued that even this distinction between the medical and social models is unnecessarily limiting because both medical treatment and social accommodation play important roles in disability experiences. They argue that, if held exclusively, each model shuts out the complexity of living with a disability and thus fails to ameliorate the experience, arguably one of the important aims of this area of engaged scholarship.[19] To the extent that engagement and activism have been central to DS, its scholars suggest, their result has at times been a sidelining of medical expertise.

Comics can play a powerful role in DS by framing disability as an experience that may include but also frequently transcends the medical context. As cartoonist Will Eisner has taught us, comics rely on the "expressive anatomy" of the body.[20] Gesture constitutes a crucial part of the comics lexicon, according to Eisner, enabling the vivid expression of human emotion coupled with the experience of specific embodiment: "[T]he human form and the language of its bodily movements become one of the essential ingredients of comic strip art."[21] In Eisner's view, the movements, posture, and gestures of the body take precedence over the words in a text, framing how we are to understand them and distilling meaning compactly and efficiently. Because comics direct our attention to the meaning conveyed by the body and its movements, gestures, and postures—even if the textual narrative may be conveying another (and conflicting) meaning—graphic medicine is able to incorporate the representations of medical treatment or the experiences of disability without framing the narrative or protagonist entirely within that category.

Kaisa Leka's *I Am Not These Feet* is a classic articulation of comics' capacity to address the experience of disability by transcending restrictive categories for disability experience.[22] This self-published black-and-white comic tells the story of the author's decision to have her congenitally arthritic feet amputated and to be fitted with foot prostheses. The comic is structured as a journal, with a date and a comment introducing each page. Beginning with a panel showing Kaisa *in utero*, captioned "Why my old feet sucked," this autobiographical comic portrays iconic experiences of medicine and disability without being framed (and thus limited) by them. Kaisa experiences "self-loathing [that] was really tearing [her] apart." Frustrated by her "stupid malformed freaky feet," she is dogged by the notion that her disability was a punishment, "God's sick joke." Indeed, she has internalized the toxic identity enforced by her normate society, and "the (seemingly) happy, healthy and pretty images of women that the media is bombarding us with. Being unhappy, sick and ugly is synonymous with failure." She makes the decision to have her legs amputated below the knee as an alternative to increasing reliance on inadequate painkillers that don't help her severe arthritis, and she enters the hospital for surgery followed by nine weeks of recovery and rehabilitation.

During this stay the experiences she encounters are central to both medical humanities and disability studies. She must run the informed consent gauntlet ("Everyone at the hospital thinks I'm mad," and "Are you sure you want to do this?"). She suffers the side effects of her medication, is saddled with a nurse unwilling to administer painkillers when she needs them, and must endure the "degrading" experience of the urinary catheter. But the comic's central focus is the period following her surgery, as it offers a fine-grained and highly embodied account of Kaisa's experience adjusting to her new prosthetic feet and relearning how to use a crutch, then to use a wheelchair, and finally to walk and run.

As Kaisa begins using her prostheses, the comic increasingly reveals her complex embodiment, showing us the adaptive and visualization technologies with which she builds her new sense of self in the world. Kaisa reveals the material objects and practices she must master in order to live with her specific disability, using a variety of strategies to shape the very space of the comics page: six tiered panels, splash pages, pages filled with speech bubbles, a full-page cutaway diagram of her prosthetic foot, and a white page whose dotted line traces the fifty-meter route she walked when she first tried crutches with her prostheses. Each panel/page shows us an action or object in its specific space and time, along with date-stamped commentary. We see the process of binding the stump properly ("Keep this in mind the next time you're amputated"), the inflatable prosthesis that is used to apply pressure to her stumps, the wheelchair she learns to maneuver thanks to tips from her friend, the space of the physiotherapy room in which she strides between the guide rails on her inflatable prostheses, and the slick carbon fiber limbs on which she will learn to walk (prostheses she will not cover with the orange plastic deceptively called "skin colored").

Then, in a sudden shift of scale and seriousness, the sequence skids from realism to synecdoche. The next panel figures a large building with a smoking chimney labeled "Waste Disposal, Inc." The caption reads, "I'm no longer ashamed of being disabled. It's as if the shame has been burnt away with my feet." The panel summons and sweeps away the memory of her amputated and discarded feet. Not only has Kaisa incorporated her new prostheses ("a part of me now"), but she also declares a new identity ("I'm a graphic designer and a comic artist"). *I Am Not These Feet* shows us that the process of adapting to a disability can enhance both flexibility and vitality, if we understand the medical context as helpful rather than constraining or determinative. The comic also enacts the ways in which new technologies can increase the communicative power of movement and gesture.

Women's Studies

"The personal is political" has been the implicit message of many works of graphic medicine that speak to the experiences of women. The expressive power of these works frequently arises in the teasing combination of hide/reveal that comics' reliance on word and image makes possible. To take one well-known example, in Marjane Satrapi's *Embroideries* the terms "graphic" and "medicine" both operate under ambiguous erasure.[23] "Embroideries" alludes to the medical procedure of vaginal suture, or hymenoplasty, that some Iranian women secretly undergo in order to satisfy their culture's fetish of female virginity. With that meaning of "embroideries" hidden in plain sight, the narrative plays with the word's alternate meanings: both the decorous feminine skills of the sewing circle and the discursive creativity on display in those hidden gatherings, where women tell frank, graphic, and even exaggerated stories of their bodily and sexual lives. The title's triple entendre unites *Embroideries*, moving us from "Prologue" (in cross-stitched title) to "Embroideries" (a cross-stitched handkerchief in embroidery hoop), through increasingly bawdy stories and images, until the seemingly orthodox seamstresses confront that most unorthodox type of embroidery: elective hymenoplasty to surgically reconstruct a woman's virginity. As Satrapi's grandmother tells her friend, Azzi, "If you miss your virginity so much, you just have to have an embroidery!"

Another kind of conversation around sexuality has served as a catalyst for a graphic medicine activist project in sex education, until recently a neglected part of the medical world.[24] *Not Your Mother's Meatloaf* (*NYMM*), a sex-ed 'zine pioneered by Liza Bley and Saiya Miller, has the motto "Experiences, not answers." True to its motto, *NYMM* accepts submissions of autobiographical or biographical comics that narrate sexual experiences. These comics were published, usually anonymously, in thematically organized issues: "Firsts," "Bodies," "Health," and "Age." The comics vary in graphic skill, some polished and others amateurish, but all of them are raw in the best sense, educating the reader by sharing significant sexual experiences rather than providing expert answers.

NYMM's practice of writing, collecting, and publishing comics about sex is at its core a project of feminist activism. Bley and Miller have written that their "primary focus is educating youth and each other about important issues surrounding sexuality, safer sex, consent, gender, etc."[25] Their website records the sex-ed workshops they have held around the country.[26] Individual issues of the comic are sold online and at feminist bookshops. Miller has also presented on *NYMM* at the International Graphic Medicine conferences in Chicago (2011) and Toronto (2012) to educate healthcare practitioners about this effective mode of sex education. The publication of *NYMM* by Soft Skull Press in 2013 took the editors on a national book tour, during which they continued to hold activist workshops as well as talks on their volume.[27] Incorporating the energy of contemporary gender and sexuality studies, with its focus on girlhood, LGBTQA sexuality, and recovery from sexual abuse—as well as the autobiographical emphasis that has been a strong feminist strategy since the early years of the women's movement—*NYMM* shares with narrative medicine an interest in the power of autobiography. As Saiya Miller explained to me in an interview I conducted with her in May 2011, "Personal narratives humanize and offer a different kind of access to our questions on sex and sexuality than the sterilized, clinical speak of most sex ed. curriculum. Comic format also catalyzes a different way of accessing and sharing information. Having a variety of resources, and presenting information in different formats, helps youth envision alternatives, sparks discussions, and acts as a template for storytelling."[28]

Miller's implication is clear: graphic medicine offers a good alternative mode of teaching sex ed. Rather than the normalizing and prescriptive mode of sex-ed curricula offered in medical or religious institutions, the comics in *NYMM* offer a plurality of sexual orientations, experiences, fantasies, and encounters with a shared emphasis on self-respect, safety, and nonjudgmental attitudes—just what the original authors of *Our Bodies, Ourselves* might have embraced.[29] Although the *DSM-5* no longer includes the diagnostic category for homosexuality,[30] a medical emphasis on sexual normativity still lingers, and works of graphic medicine offer important alternatives to it. In its emancipatory energy, *NYMM* belongs on the Queer Theory bookshelf right alongside comics that testify more acutely to the pains and pleasures of growing up non-normative in a normate culture, like Alison Bechdel's *Fun Home* and Ariel Schrag's *Potential*.

Science and Technology Studies and Environmental Studies

One of the core concepts in science and technology studies is the notion that technologies configure their users. Taken more broadly still, this notion reveals that things have agency: they can act on, and even act back at, the people who use them, shaping processes and outcomes. The significant social implications of this concept make both science and technology studies (STS) and environmental studies active sites of engaged scholarship. Science studies scholars study the networks of relationships linking things and people in order to learn the processes by which scientific facts are produced, to affirm the importance of strong objectivity in scientific practice, and to shape a more just and equitable science and society.

Environmental studies scholars often also adapt the actor-network approach to link environmental phenomena (such as a chemical spill) to the people and institutions upstream and downstream—both temporally and spatially—from the chemical production process. The volume of medical issues addressed by STS and environmental studies increases daily, as the wicked problems of contemporary life exceed any tidy epistemological and disciplinary categorizations. Ken Dahl's *Monsters* addresses this complex area of concern, in which issues of medicine are inextricably linked to issues of science, technology, and the environment.[31]

Monsters tells the story of Ken, whose fear of transmitting herpes—nourished by scary information from the medical and online worlds—inhibits his personal relationships with women. The comic follows Ken's reaction to the shock of discovering that he is infected, as he attempts to adjust to the herpes he believes he carries and to escape his status as celibate pariah. We watch as the same medical and informatics technologies that aim to control herpes also spread it as a node of iatrogenically caused anxiety and a stigmatized identity. Herpes morphs into a set of emotionally laden social-technical networks: the TV commercials for Valtrex, whose happy, laughing, herpes-infected actors Ken scorns as inconsiderate and irresponsible (5); the blood test through which Ken and his girlfriend learn the shocking news that they have both tested positive for the herpes simplex virus (29); and, most of all, the internet search for herpes images that serves up contagion stories "like something out of a monster movie" (51–53). In a sequence of pages whose images recall *Frankenstein*—that classic text for science studies—as well as images of industrial degradation familiar to environmental studies, Ken confronts his own monstrosity (55–58). Like all monsters, he yearns for "what everyone else wants—acceptance; affection; inclusion . . . and of course, survival" (55). And yet the page reveals that his survival is really threatened not by herpes but by its social and environmental context. A splash page pictures the torch-wielding, monster-hunting villagers from *Frankenstein*. As they march across a bridge, shouting "Kill! Kill! Kill!," a monstrous Ken walks miserably beneath them, through the refuse-laden water, past a sign that warns: "No Fishing: Mercury Advisory" (58). The social stigma of herpes revealed on the bridge above is mirrored by the toxic environment below.

Community building is a central strategy of graphic medicine. Thus, the autobiographical narrative of *Monsters* pauses to bring the reader into the story by using direct address, revealing that Ken is not the only pariah. The section titled "Herpes A brief and confusing introduction"—an X-rated remix of *Little Nemo* and *In the Night Kitchen*[32]—reveals a naked Ken tumbling through a nightmare flood of information on herpes. Frightening images accompany the text: the virus's life cycle; the "Wheel O' Transmission," by which the virus moves through a population;

the distinctions between the benign Type 1 and the "dirty" Type 2 viruses; and, most terrifying of all, an anatomical atlas of all the places on the body where herpes can manifest itself in an almost biblical array of scourges (108–19). Later, an Adamic man and an Eve-like woman manifest the phenomenon of "asymptomatic viral shedding" (116). The information provided moves from comprehensive to exhaustive and finally to exhausting, at which point a naked Ken, tumbling between virions larger than his head, puts it all together for us: "You can get herpes from pretty much ANYONE . . . at pretty much any TIME . . . on pretty much any part of your BODY? . . . Why did no one ever TELL me about any of this?" (117–18).

The comic does not give Ken's catastrophism the last word, however. After trying out scores of alternative treatments for herpes and braving the horrors of online dating, Ken finally meets a girl able to put his worries into perspective: "I can't believe out of all the things in the world to obsess over, you chose THIS! Sure, herpes can be embarrassing, and maybe even uncomfortable, but COME ON . . . It's a SKIN RASH! And it goes away. There's even drugs to suppress it now!" (189). Ken, morphed into a herpes pustule, replies, "I'm just trying to be safe" (189). When she retorts, "Look, I know there's a chance—an EXTREMELY SMALL chance—that you can still transmit herpes even when you're not having an outbreak . . . And I'm actually flattered that you'd even think to TELL me . . . But . . . Well . . . Don't be such a WUSS!" (190), she finally reaches him. The herpes pustule engulfing him ruptures, and Ken emerges, exclaiming, "I feel like I've been waiting years for someone to say that" (191).

Ken and his herpes virus reach a détente in a conversation that is the comic's "Epilogue": "Even if you never have an outbreak," the virus tells Ken, "we're still with you for the rest of your life" (198). And Ken muses, "Why was I so MESSED UP about it? It's like five years of my life were just a corny sex-ed PSA" (199). The virus sums it up for both of them: "I'm just another life form trying to survive in this weird, fucked-up world" (200). In this final image, Ken and his herpes muse companionably on the same bridge over which had marched the mob of angry villagers; Frankenstein's monster has become Frankenstein's "little buddy." In its final vision of that polluted river, *Monsters* links the biomedical and environmental strategies by which we simultaneously manage and maintain our risk society.[33] Dahl's contribution to graphic medicine joins *NYMM* as an example of an activist form of sex ed and medical education, informing its readers and enabling them to gain some measure of emotional control over the atmosphere of risk assessment that suffuses daily life.

Graphic Medicine Further Afield

Works in graphic medicine also have the potential to raise urgent questions often neglected in several other significant areas of scholarly research and teaching.

Scholars in postcolonial studies can turn to works of graphic medicine to explore the effects of alternative medical practices in a Western medical environment (*Epileptic*, by David B.) or the medical effects of racism and/or war in both developed and "developing" nations (*Level Up* by Gene Luen Yang and Thien Pham and *American Born Chinese* by Gene Luen Yang and Lark Pien, as well as *Deogratias: A Story of Rwanda* by Jean-Philippe Stassen). Animal studies scholars will be drawn to the powerful portrayal of animal military-and-medical testing and suffering in *We3*; the image of a contagious, disease-producing trans-species transformation in *Ode to Kirihito*; and the unmistakable depression and anxiety experienced by industrial chickens threatened with the slaughterhouse in *Elmer*.[34] They may also find works of graphic medicine to be productive texts with which to explore the overlap between veterinary and human medicine.[35]

Even before the veterinary-human medicine convergence occurs, we are likely to find the publication of new works of graphic veterinary medicine—*pet-pathographies*, if you will—which may be aimed at educating veterinarians or pet owners or which may testify to the illness experiences of the animal patients or their caregivers. By extending pathographies beyond the human, healthcare personnel beyond physicians and nurses to family members, patients, and the population more broadly, and sources for meaningful health-related communication beyond literary texts to the fields of visual and popular culture, the medical humanities field has developed into a widely suggestive program for critical health studies.

Graphic Medicine in the Graduate Classroom

Later contributors to this volume detail the many ways in which graphic medicine can enrich the perspectives of the medical student, healthcare worker, nurse, or physician during the clinical encounter. For most of my career, in contrast, I have been teaching people whose primary relationship to the medical experience is as a patient, a relative of a patient, or a caregiver. Graphic medicine clearly has value in that it broadens each individual's resources for dealing with illness, medicine, and disability. However, since I write this in the context of what some are calling a "crisis in the humanities"[36]—but which is, to my thinking, rather an exciting opportunity to revitalize our work as humanities scholars and teachers—I want to close by exploring how graphic medicine can invigorate the graduate classroom in the humanities and perhaps even graduate work writ large.

I have been arguing that graphic medicine can inform engaged scholarship in a number of different research areas in the humanities. Yet if we are adding graphic medicine to the syllabus in doctoral courses in the humanities, we first need to know how to teach comics to our graduate students. This can pose some challenges. Consider, for example, the training for an English Ph.D. It instills crucial skills for the professional job market: critical acumen, linguistic fluency, competition, and a drive for mastery. These qualities can actually be handicaps for someone interested in learning about a new art form, however. Caution and careerism can inhibit a student trying to experiment with different modes of perception and expression. Graduate students must face the fact that the literary canon until very recently has had very little room for comics, and they must find an answer to the perennial question of critical methodology: what analytical tools can they use to study this new medium? The bottom line can be discouragement: why should students spend their time writing about comics when there seems to be little professional payoff?

As Scott Smith has pointed out, these questions have a certain history already in the realm of comics studies, where for some the answer has been to repeat the same critical and theoretical moves that English literature scholars have always used: to argue the aesthetic, philosophical, and thematic significance, the rigor, and the value of the comic as a work of art. And yet . . . the mask of the critic is too brittle to be expressive. The lifeblood oozes out of the vibrant form that is graphic medicine when it is pressed into the standard literary-critical mold. To be useful for engaged scholarship, comics criticism needs to make connections beyond the university and even let some urgency slip into its tone. We need to train our graduate students to do comics studies on its own terms, rather than as a pallid version of literary criticism.

The answer, I believe, is to learn something about the process of making comics. So, I incorporate studio time into my English department doctoral seminars on graphic narrative. True, the thought of trying to draw can be frightening to students trained to write and read texts. As someone who has learned to think of myself as a verbal rather than visual person, I empathize with this fear. Yet as MK Czerwiec details later in this volume, Lynda Barry's work provides a vigorous challenge to the notion that visual skills are inherent. And if I'm willing to learn something about drawing comics in order to shake myself open to this new medium, I can persuade my students that they, too, should have some skin in the game. The benefits are many. Students may have entered the classroom a little sheepish about reading "for credit" works that, for years, they may have been reading on the sly, scorning as not literary, or simply avoiding as not to their taste. Yet whether the students are hardcore comics enthusiasts or wary neophytes, this period of "studio time" seems to enable them to shrug off their discomfort, turn off their knee-jerk mechanism of critique for a while, and open themselves to the new medium.

The studio structure is simple. During the first hour of the seminar, we typically discuss the comic(s) assigned for that class meeting, focusing on plot, imagery, graphic structure, and narrative strategies; we discuss the analytic evaluative responses the students present in their assigned response papers, which we will return to in the third hour. But in the middle, we do an hour of studio practice during which all of us—students as well as professor—draw comics. We have a text to guide us; most recently I have chosen either Ivan Brunetti's *Cartooning: Philosophy and Practice* or Jessica Abel and Matt Madden's *Drawing Words and Writing Pictures*. This semester—as I write this chapter—I have also put Robyn Chapman's *Drawing Comics Lab* on course reserve.[37] Often we'll have a guest. For example, cartoonist Jarod Roselló has co-taught the studio portion of the class, introducing students to some of the basics of comics creation: drawing the face and the body, paneling, building tiers, composing a plot in word and image, and shaping the final product, four-page comics of the students' own creation.[38] Jay Hosler, Frank Ottaviani, Alison Bechdel, Ian Williams, MK Czerwiec, Michael Green, and Joyce Farmer have all appeared as stimulating guest speakers, sharing their respective experiences with science cartooning, comics scripting, page layout, and the use of reference photos, as well as the strategies for teaching comics making to medical school students.

As the studio portion of the class progresses through the semester, I sometimes have to tinker with my approaches, depending on the composition of the class. One semester, I had several students who were very familiar with drawing as well as others who were relaxed enough to enjoy the novelty of the activity; another semester I had students whose critical proclivities leaned toward philosophy and theory, which made the act of drawing, rather than writing, highly challenging. In that case, we began by making a jam comic, a popular strategy for introducing the creation of comics to people who have never drawn. Starting with a piece of paper gridded into nine panels, three in a row, each student is asked to write a story by captioning every panel; they then illustrate the first panel (based on the caption), and pass it to the student on the left.[39] The next person draws the second panel, passes it to the left, and so on, until the nine panels are filled. (This process may be familiar to graduate students working in literary modernism who have encountered the surrealist game Exquisite Corpse.) The result of this nine-person collaboration is a one-page, nine-panel comic whose panels and captions collide in unexpected and wonderful ways.[40] This relaxes students and breaks the ice; then the individual drawing process begins.[41]

My goal for the studio time has never been to produce cartoonists, although by the semester's end nearly all of the students will have taken the extra-credit option and produced their own four-page comic. Some students have gone on to produce minicomics, while one student collaborated with his cartoonist brother to create a web comic on diabetes.[42] However, I want to focus on using the cartooning process to enhance the students' skills as readers of comics and to improve the comics scholarship they will write. I hope to create two specific changes in their work.

First, I want them to learn to focus in their writing less on critique and more on concern. Let me explain what I mean by this. In an essay published in 2003, science studies scholar Bruno Latour asked, "Can we devise another powerful descriptive tool that deals this time with matters of concern and whose import then will no longer be to debunk but to protect and to care, as Donna Haraway would put it? . . . Is it really possible to solve the question, to write not matter-of-factually but, how should I say it, in a matter-of-concern way?"[43] Latour was addressing the science wars, when the concept of social construction—the core tenet of science studies for decades—was adapted by the anti-science reactionary right to challenge scientifically accepted notions such as global climate change. His insight was that the habit of criticism, which had given us such powerful analytic and deconstructive techniques, began to work against the emancipatory hopes of science studies. The conservative right soon learned to deploy these critical tools in order to challenge important scientific findings from their own perspective, replacing scientific truth with "truthiness." Latour argued in response that we should move beyond the academic habit of detached critique and instead "associate the word *criticism* with a whole set of new positive metaphors, gestures, attitudes, knee-jerk reactions, habits of thoughts" (247).

While Latour's reason for advocating an alternative to critique lay in his dismay at the declining public understanding of science, mine lies in the wish to increase the public understanding of humanities scholarship. Nonetheless, we share the sense that critique has become too easy and perhaps ineffective. What is hard and important, if perhaps a bit embarrassing, is to speak to issues of concern: issues that move us, inspire us, and make us want to take action. The difficulty, pride, and satisfaction of learning how to create in the comics medium—what we had hitherto just been reading and critiquing—was my goal for the studio hour. The activism might follow.

In some of the meetings of the comics seminars that I have taught so far, the studio experience did seem to have that effect; the literature scholars-in-the-making sloughed off their sophistication temporarily to become novice cartoonists. After struggling to draw a face, or fit text into a panel, or represent movement, they found themselves increasingly reluctant to dismiss a work with scorn (a fairly familiar graduate student attitude). They felt increasingly willing to participate imaginatively in the structure, plot, image, and organizational choices of the comics they were reading, because they understood some of the challenges the cartoonist might have been facing. They reminded me of the new community of critics Latour invokes with passion: "The critic is not the one who debunks, but the one who assembles. The critic is not the one who lifts the rugs from under the feet of the naïve believers, but the one who offers the participants arenas in which to gather" (246).

My second aim is to help my students improve their revision skills. The process of thumbnailing an entire comic after the script is drafted—sketching in rough versions of each page—can be both illuminating and humbling. It requires students to think spatially as well as temporally, to bring the synchronic and diachronic aspects of narrative together, improving their narrative skills in both dimensions. Thumbnailing also teaches students that their stories aren't "tellable" in the form they had initially selected. Forced to shift focus, change the order of the plot, even remove or revise characters or events because the comics medium demands it, students often discover the heart of the story, producing comics with an intensity and focus their first versions had lacked.[44] For students working in the humanities—who need to learn to write prose compelling to an audience extending beyond their academic peers, because the incorporation of a wider audience is not only educationally sound but politically imperative within and beyond the university—the study of graphic medicine is a valuable tool.

A Postscript on Caring

I found that including graphic medicine as part of studio time in the comics classroom helped my text-focused English Ph.D. students care about the form and content of comics. It did much more than that, however. As we worked our way through the elements of making comics—learning about paneling, speech balloons, emanata, gutters, tiers, and splash pages—the students' engagement with the comics medium was initially rather superficial. Making their first comics, they played with a range of genres—superhero, whimsical animals, talking heads, evil monsters—in a mood more casual, playful, and detached than the one they customarily use in their written literary scholarship. But the mood in the classroom changed noticeably when I mentioned that they could choose an issue linked to medicine, illness, or disability for their four-page final comics, and they began to create comics about a medical experience, whether their own or one of a parent, sibling, or friend. They cared about representing those experiences effectively, and they created those comics with absorption and pleasure. Even though this was a graduate seminar in English, rather than a course in the medical humanities, and even though they were working on creating their own comics rather than discussing classic literary texts, they acquired the intellectual and emotional tools central to the field of narrative medicine, tools that enabled them, as Rita Charon has put it, "to take these multiple, contradictory narratives, and let them build something that we can act on."[45] And that's a pretty powerful expression of the uses of graphic medicine for engaged scholarship.

· · · · · · · · ·

I chose the following excerpts from comics because they have been major influences on my uses of comics in research and teaching: Ruben Bolling's "Bad Blastocyst," a one-page syncretic comic riff on the multiple ways bioethics, politics, and the law can engage with the field of embryo research; Kaisa Leka's *I Am*

Not These Feet, a remarkable homage to the "funny animals" tradition in comics, as well as its darker undercurrent, which transforms the cute, iconic, and universal into the powerfully pragmatic and specific; and Ann Starr's "Where Babies Come From: A Miracle Explained," a satire of the medical information pamphlet as feminist autography.[46] They also suggest the remarkable breadth of comics as a medium, incorporating not only the syndicated comic strip but also the handmade, one-of-a-kind minicomic and the self-published graphic pathography later reissued by a commercial press.

FIGURES ON
FOLLOWING PAGES
▬ ▬ ▬ ▬ ▬ ▬

fig. 2.2
Ruben Bolling, "Bad Blastocyst." From Bolling, *Thrilling Tom the Dancing Bug Stories: A Collection of the Weekly Comic Strip "Tom the Dancing Bug"* (Kansas City, MO: Andrews McMeel, 2004).

figs. 2.3–2.5
From Kaisa Leka, *I Am Not These Feet* (Helsinki: Absolute Truth Press, 2008).

figs. 2.6–2.7
From Ann Starr, "Where Babies Come From: A Miracle Explained," artist's book, 1997.

fig. 2.2

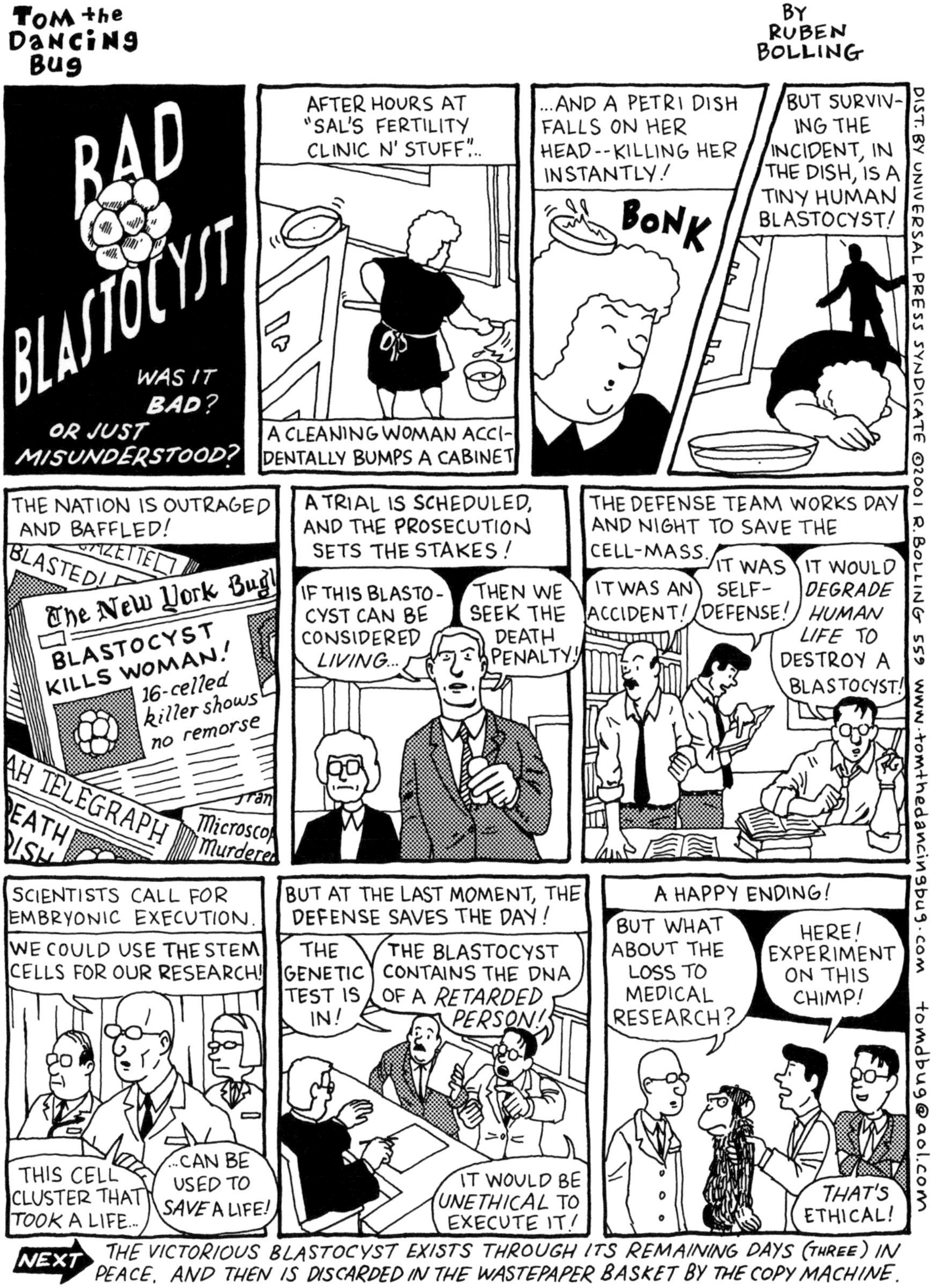

TOM the DANCING BUG
BY RUBEN BOLLING
BAD BLASTOCYST
WAS IT BAD? OR JUST MISUNDERSTOOD?
AFTER HOURS AT "SAL'S FERTILITY CLINIC N' STUFF"...
A CLEANING WOMAN ACCIDENTALLY BUMPS A CABINET
...AND A PETRI DISH FALLS ON HER HEAD--KILLING HER INSTANTLY!
BONK
BUT SURVIVING THE INCIDENT, IN THE DISH, IS A TINY HUMAN BLASTOCYST!
THE NATION IS OUTRAGED AND BAFFLED!
BLASTED!
The New York Bugl
BLASTOCYST KILLS WOMAN!
16-celled killer shows no remorse
AH TELEGRAPH
DEATH DISH
Microscop Murderer
A TRIAL IS SCHEDULED, AND THE PROSECUTION SETS THE STAKES!
IF THIS BLASTOCYST CAN BE CONSIDERED LIVING...
THEN WE SEEK THE DEATH PENALTY!
THE DEFENSE TEAM WORKS DAY AND NIGHT TO SAVE THE CELL-MASS.
IT WAS AN ACCIDENT!
IT WAS SELF-DEFENSE!
IT WOULD DEGRADE HUMAN LIFE TO DESTROY A BLASTOCYST!
SCIENTISTS CALL FOR EMBRYONIC EXECUTION.
WE COULD USE THE STEM CELLS FOR OUR RESEARCH!
THIS CELL CLUSTER THAT TOOK A LIFE...
...CAN BE USED TO SAVE A LIFE!
BUT AT THE LAST MOMENT, THE DEFENSE SAVES THE DAY!
THE GENETIC TEST IS IN!
THE BLASTOCYST CONTAINS THE DNA OF A RETARDED PERSON!
IT WOULD BE UNETHICAL TO EXECUTE IT!
A HAPPY ENDING!
BUT WHAT ABOUT THE LOSS TO MEDICAL RESEARCH?
HERE! EXPERIMENT ON THIS CHIMP!
THAT'S ETHICAL!
DIST. BY UNIVERSAL PRESS SYNDICATE ©2001 R. BOLLING 559 www.tomthedancingbug.com tomdbug@aol.com
NEXT THE VICTORIOUS BLASTOCYST EXISTS THROUGH ITS REMAINING DAYS (THREE) IN PEACE. AND THEN IS DISCARDED IN THE WASTEPAPER BASKET BY THE COPY MACHINE.

fig. 2.3

MONDAY MARCH 18TH, 2002
I'M LUCKY TO HAVE A GREAT PROSTHETIST

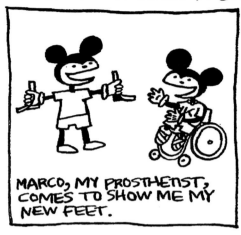

MARCO, MY PROSTHETIST, COMES TO SHOW ME MY NEW FEET.

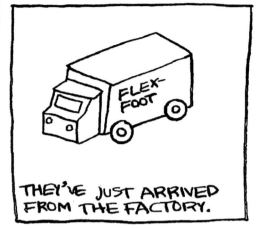

THEY'VE JUST ARRIVED FROM THE FACTORY.

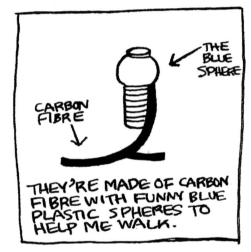

THE BLUE SPHERE

CARBON FIBRE

THEY'RE MADE OF CARBON FIBRE WITH FUNNY BLUE PLASTIC SPHERES TO HELP ME WALK.

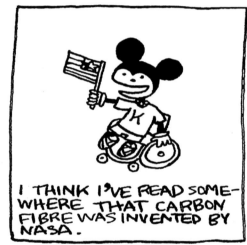

I THINK I'VE READ SOME-WHERE THAT CARBON FIBRE WAS INVENTED BY NASA.

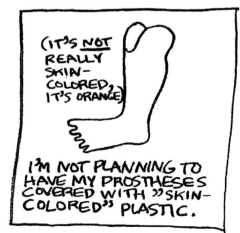

(IT'S NOT REALLY SKIN-COLORED, IT'S ORANGE)

I'M NOT PLANNING TO HAVE MY PROSTHESES COVERED WITH "SKIN-COLORED" PLASTIC.

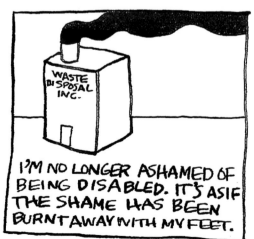

WASTE DISPOSAL INC.

I'M NO LONGER ASHAMED OF BEING DISABLED. IT'S AS IF THE SHAME HAS BEEN BURNT AWAY WITH MY FEET.

fig. 2.4

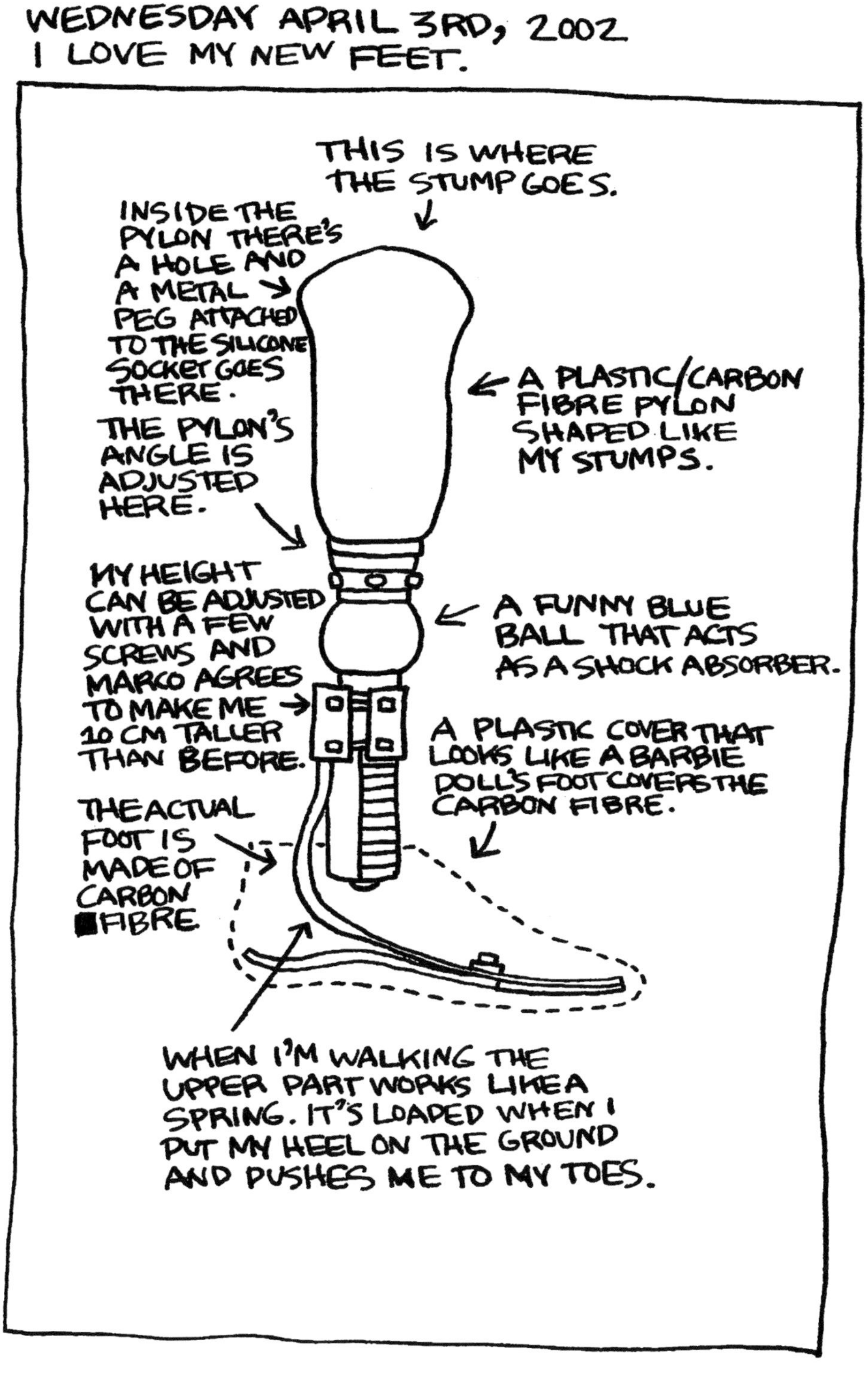

WEDNESDAY APRIL 3RD, 2002
I LOVE MY NEW FEET.
THIS IS WHERE THE STUMP GOES.
INSIDE THE PYLON THERE'S A HOLE AND A METAL PEG ATTACHED TO THE SILICONE SOCKET GOES THERE.
A PLASTIC/CARBON FIBRE PYLON SHAPED LIKE MY STUMPS.
THE PYLON'S ANGLE IS ADJUSTED HERE.
MY HEIGHT CAN BE ADJUSTED WITH A FEW SCREWS AND MARCO AGREES TO MAKE ME 10 CM TALLER THAN BEFORE.
A FUNNY BLUE BALL THAT ACTS AS A SHOCK ABSORBER.
A PLASTIC COVER THAT LOOKS LIKE A BARBIE DOLL'S FOOT COVERS THE CARBON FIBRE.
THE ACTUAL FOOT IS MADE OF CARBON FIBRE
WHEN I'M WALKING THE UPPER PART WORKS LIKE A SPRING. IT'S LOADED WHEN I PUT MY HEEL ON THE GROUND AND PUSHES ME TO MY TOES.

fig. 2.5

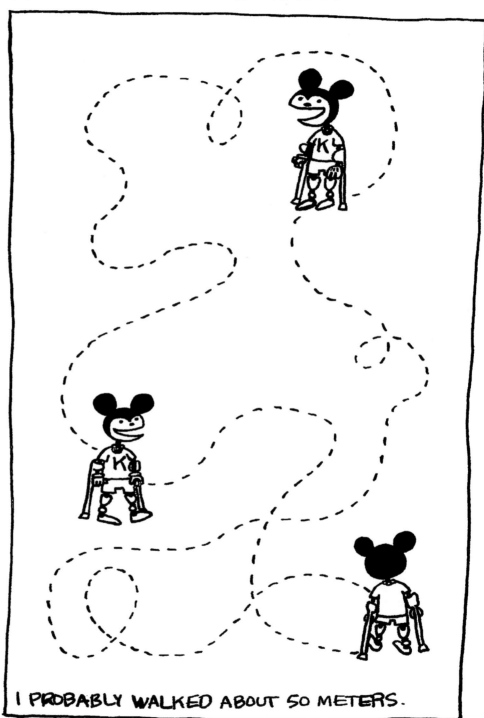

THURSDAY APRIL 4TH, 2002
I'M WALKING WITH CRUTCHES!

I PROBABLY WALKED ABOUT 50 METERS.

fig. 2.6

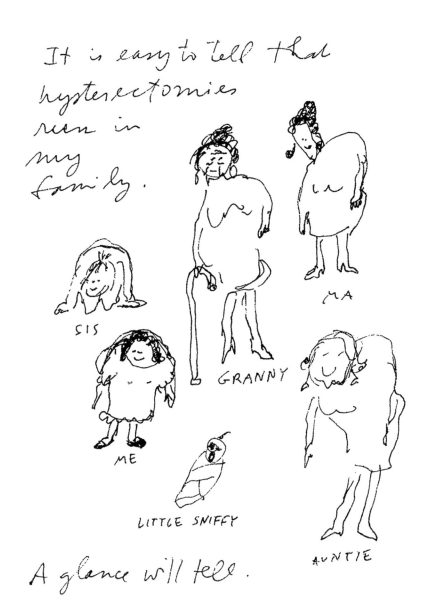

It is easy to tell that
hysterectomies
run in
my
family.

SIS

GRANNY

MA

ME

LITTLE SNIFFY

AUNTIE

A glance will tell.

fig. 2.7

None of us have any sex organs.
* enlargement!
nothing. zip. rien.
ON
REPRESENTATIVE OF THE FAMILY

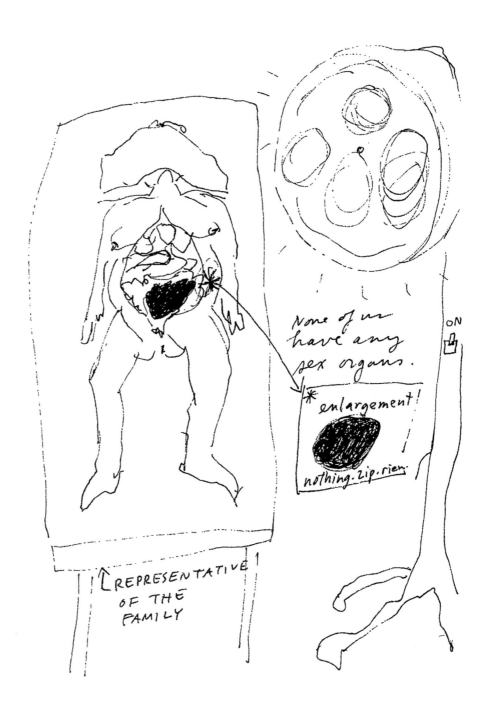

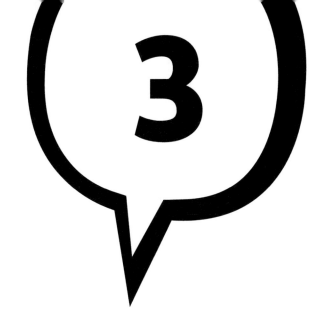

Graphic Storytelling and Medical Narrative

The Use of Comics in Medical Education

- - - - -

Michael J. Green

Introduction

When one thinks about medical education, what typically comes to mind are the intense memorization of basic sciences, dissection in the gross anatomy lab, long and arduous work hours, and rotation through myriad clinical specialties. Much has been written about the ritualistic hazing and indoctrination into this gilded profession and how students are transformed from novices to experts through apprenticeship, trial and error, and mere survival (hence the joke: "What do you call a medical student who graduates last in his class? Answer: Doctor").

In the vast literature on medical education, one would be hard pressed to find mention of graphic novels or comics, as medical educators are apt to associate this medium with frivolousness, juvenile fantasies, or caped superheroes who simply have no place in a serious medical school curriculum. Nevertheless, in this chapter, I will describe how graphic narratives (or comics[1]) can be (and have been) integrated into medical education, as well as a role they can serve in the curriculum. While my comments refer to teaching medical students, they could just as well apply to the education of other healthcare professionals, but since my experience is within a medical school, I will focus on the medical-student population.

My Origin Story

I suppose I have always been "into" comics—something of which I was reminded while cleaning my basement as I waited for Hurricane Sandy to strike central Pennsylvania. Trying to prevent the storm from damaging my valuables, I discovered an old portfolio of my childhood school activities and artwork, including a third-grade report on the life cycle of termites. Though I didn't know it at the time, I had created a comic. While the other children dutifully drafted a paragraph or two explaining how insects live and die, I presented an illustrated tour of termite life from egg to adult. The drawings showed the story while the words filled in the gaps. My termite project received an A++++ grade, so the teacher must have liked my "comics" approach, too!

Throughout grade school, drawing was my passion, and I was considered "the artist" among my friends, winning a number of awards and scholarships for my creations. Of course, I also had the obligatory comic book collection while growing up. I particularly liked *The Fantastic Four* and *Spider-Man*[2]—I suppose I related to the alienated outsider aspect of the characters—and I spent many afternoons reading these adventures. But as an older child and young adult, I didn't really spend much time or energy thinking about comics, and I donated my meager collection to my younger brother as I moved on to more "mature" interests.

Fast forward to college. During my sophomore year, I briefly toyed with the idea of becoming a medical illustrator. I relished the idea of combining my sympathy for science with my ardor for art. I loved to draw (still do) and to tell stories with my drawings. I thought medical illustration would let me do just that. But in the end, I decided to apply to medical school, as I wanted the human interaction that doctoring required—and I didn't like the idea of having a bunch of physicians telling me what to draw.

In medical school, my favorite study materials were *The Anatomy Coloring Book* and *Clinical Neuroanatomy Made Ridiculously Simple*, both books that provided simple but informative drawings to explain complex medical concepts.[3] To study, I would construct images of nerve pathways, muscle function, and kidney tubules in an effort to understand visually how the body was supposed to work when it wasn't ravaged by disease. While I wasn't quite embarrassed by my books and learning methods, I didn't make these study habits known to my classmates, who I worried would find such materials to be too rudimentary for the medical school classroom. Even so, they got me through the courses, I learned the material, and I enjoyed studying in my own way.

I graduated from medical school, completed a residency program in internal medicine, trained as a bioethicist, and secured a faculty position in the Department of Humanities at Penn State College of Medicine. Though comics played no role in my early years as a faculty member, Penn State offered opportunities that were a perfect fit for my varied interests. Indeed, Penn State has a proud history of introducing many curricular innovations into medical education—including the distinction of having established the first Department of Humanities in any U.S. medical school. So I developed a variety of nontraditional courses for medical students, such as seminars on medical ethics at the movies and literature on the medical wards. While such courses were interesting and rewarding, after a while, I began to feel that something was missing. The students and I talked about and interpreted the works of others, and we applied humanities disciplines to medicine, but we didn't create anything new. I wanted to truly merge the arts with the sciences, but I needed to figure out a way to make that happen.

Then I started to read comics again. I discovered Art Spiegelman's *Maus* and was astounded to learn that serious and important topics could be presented using the comic format. I read Will Eisner's *A Contract With God* and began to ponder the use of comics for exploring ethical issues. I devoured Charles Burns's *Black Hole* and saw how medical themes could be integrated into a graphic narrative. The idea for a course on comics for medical students emerged, and I began to seriously consider ways to use this material in medical education.

Figuring that there would be no point in reinventing the wheel, I contacted colleagues at other institutions and searched online to see who else was using comics in medical education. I soon learned that no one was doing this—if it was going to happen, I would need to concoct such a course myself. So I started to pull together resources (at which time I stumbled upon Ian Williams's newly created Graphic Medicine website[4]), and I developed the first-ever course on comics and medicine for medical students.

Why Comics?

For many years, educators have relied on myriad forms of literature to expose medical students to various aspects of the illness experience. Novels, short stories, poems, and plays about medical topics illuminate the social and cultural context of sickness, expose students to the emotions intertwined with illness, and help prepare students for a life beyond the classroom.[5] Likewise, visually oriented teachers have used fine art to sharpen students' powers of observation, improve their deductive reasoning, and even promote team-building skills.[6] Though the use of comics in medical education is new, the rationale for doing so is not; teaching with comics simply applies the pedagogical goals of the older art forms to another medium. Yet because the medium combines words *and* images, it requires (and rewards) new modes of inquiry. This presents an opportunity to educate the reader in both narrative and visual literacy, skills that have relevance not only for students of medicine but for practicing physicians as well.

TABLE 3.1   SESSION TOPICS

Session	Topic
1	Why comics are relevant to medicine
2	Elements of storytelling
3	The relationship between images and words
4	Exploring point of view
5	Drawing comics
6	Writing dialogue
7	Social context of medicine
8	Final presentations

Educators in fields outside of medicine have been using comics in the classroom for more than sixty years. Even so, quantifiable data about how well they perform is scarce. Comics have been integrated into curricula as varied as college physics, business ethics, and literacy,[7] but few of these uses have been rigorously evaluated for effectiveness. One notable exception is a study by Jay Hosler and K. B. Boomer about whether comics can help students better learn and appreciate science. While not specifically dealing with medicine, this study sheds light on how one might use comics to teach traditionally challenging concepts to those who may not be open to the subject matter, or to comics, or both.[8]

Using a comic created by Hosler (*Optical Allusions*) as a course text, the researchers evaluated the impact of this book on non–science majors' attitudes and skills. Pre- and post-course data were gathered using a modified version of the Biology and Attitude Scale, a validated instrument in use for over thirty years.[9] The authors found significant increases in student knowledge as well as positive attitudes toward biology and comics at the end of the course. While not a definitive study on the impact of comics on science education, this does provide supporting evidence for the use of such materials in higher learning, and the findings mirror those from my own classroom experience with medical students.

A Course on Comics and Medicine for Medical Students

Since 2009, I have offered a popular course on comics and medicine to fourth-year medical students. Taught seminar style, in groups of eight to ten, the class meets twice weekly for four consecutive weeks. The course has two overarching objectives: (1) to teach students to *read* medically related comics critically, and (2) to help students *create* an original comic based on a meaningful medical school experience.

TABLE 3.2   SELECT GRAPHIC MEDICINE TEXTS

Title	Author	Medical topic	Summary	Year
Psychiatric Tales: Eleven Graphic Stories About Mental Illness	Darryl Cunningham	Mental illness	A series of stories about psychiatric illnesses derived from the author's experience working on a psychiatric ward.	2010
Monsters	Ken Dahl	Herpes	A man is convinced he has herpes and is tortured by anxiety, isolation, and fear as he tries to deal with the disease.	2009
Cancer Made Me a Shallower Person: A Memoir in Comics	Miriam Engelberg	Breast cancer	The author's brutally honest and often funny account of her experiences after developing breast cancer at age forty-three.	2006
Special Exits	Joyce Farmer	Aging, death and dying	A memoir chronicling the declining health of the author's parents, and the challenges of coping with the fragility of life.	2010
Disrepute	Thom Ferrier	Doctor's perspective	A physician-artist's dark look at the practice of medicine and the secret thoughts that doctors sometimes harbor.	2012
Mom's Cancer	Brian Fies	Lung cancer	The author's account of the challenges of navigating the health care system after his mother develops cancer.	2006
Marbles: Mania, Depression, Michelangelo, and Me; A Graphic Memoir	Ellen Forney	Bipolar illness	An artist struggles with her bipolar illness, debating whether treatment will dampen her creativity.	2012
Tangles: A Story About Alzheimer's, My Mother, and Me	Sarah Leavitt	Alzheimer's disease	When the author's mother develops Alzheimer's disease, the family is transformed and Sarah must figure out how to be engaged despite living far away.	2012
Years of the Elephant	Willie Linthout (trans. Michiel Horn)	Suicide, grief	A grieving father attempts to understand and cope with his son's suicide.	2009
Seeds	Ross Mackintosh	Death and dying	The author's experience of his dad's terminal illness and eventual death, told simply and lovingly.	2011
Cancer Vixen: A True Story	Marisa Acocella Marchetto	Breast cancer	A memoir of a hip, urban woman who develops breast cancer, and how she deals with the impact on her love life, personal relationships, and self-image.	2006
Stitches	David Small	Childhood cancer	The author's recollection of his unhappy childhood and what happens when he develops neck cancer and loses the ability to speak.	2009

These objectives are achieved by having students engage in three distinct activities during each class session, which lasts for two and a half hours: discussion of readings, an in-class exercise, and sharing ongoing work-in-progress toward a final comic project. Typical session topics are shown in table 3.1. Although the course readings have varied over the years, we have read part or all of each of the graphic narratives listed in table 3.2, as well as a variety of background readings on creating comics (e.g., *Making Comics*; *The Complete Idiot's Guide to Creating a Graphic Novel*; and *Drawing Words and Writing Pictures*).[10] With guidance, students are generally assigned the task of leading class discussions.

In recent years, I have arranged videoconference calls with many of the authors of these comics, providing students with an opportunity to ask questions of the artists and to glean ideas for their own projects. These fascinating conversations have been immensely popular, enabling students to obtain insights unavailable through reading alone.

In addition to discussing these books, students typically participate in an in-class exercise each session. The activities are varied and focus on helping students think creatively and without inhibitions. Toward this end, on the first day of class, I ask students to begin telling stories by having them complete "stems," such as:

- One thing about being a medical student that my family doesn't understand is . . .
- My proudest moment as a medical student was when I . . .
- I was most disappointed in myself when I . . .
- The funniest thing that I experienced as a medical student was . . .
- I was really impressed with a colleague when s/he. . . .
- One of the most troubling things I ever experienced in medicine was . . .
- I really love my work when . . .
- It was especially hard for me to deal with my patient when s/he . . .

These quick musings provide great fodder for discussion and reflection, and students split up into pairs to talk about their comments further. As homework, I assign students the task of beginning to develop one or more of these remarks into a more detailed story that might be used as the basis for their final comic project.

Other activities include lessons in drawing facial expressions, basics of storytelling, and experiments in putting words together with images. To help students practice dialogue writing, I bring to class a published comic with one alteration: all the word balloons are empty. I then ask the students to complete the story by filling the balloons with dialogue. The results are revealing not only for showing the diverse ways in which a story can be told but also for the humor and creativity that emerge through this exercise. For example, whereas one student's dialogue tells the story of a lovers' spat and dissatisfaction within a marriage, another student tells an equally convincing tale of a drug deal gone sour. By sharing and discussing their varied interpretations of sequential images, the students quickly learn how the tone, direction, and meaning of a story can be shaped through dialogue.

Reading Comics and the Curricular Goals of Medical Education

Fundamentally, medical education is concerned with teaching students how to think and act like doctors. While *thinking* emphasizes particular cognitive processes, *acting* stresses measurable skills and outcomes. Having students read carefully selected comics can further both objectives. For example, comics can be used to help students think critically and deductively, essential competencies for diagnostic reasoning. In the medical context, a physician's task is to take scattered bits of information elicited from patients' stories (the medical history) and their bodies (the physical exam) and to deduce meaning from these data to create an explanatory narrative conforming to a recognizable pattern. The physician does this despite having access to incomplete details, conflicting evidence, and distracting outliers. Yet by understanding how the body works, patterns of normal and abnormal physiology, and the language of medicine, an experienced physician can take these muddled pieces and assemble them into a coherent and meaningful narrative.

Reading comics involves a similar set of cognitive activities. By necessity, creators of comics make economical use of space and time, providing incomplete visual and written accounts. The reader must stitch together pictorial and textual clues, filling in the blank spaces between panels to determine what happened, when it occurred, and over what duration. As comics leap between time, space, and point of view, the reader must apply experience, skill, and knowledge to both complete the story and convert it into a coherent narrative. The act of reading comics critically can make explicit the processes by which the reader is an active participant in the story; this also helps students understand diagnostic reasoning, an activity that likewise involves attention to words (the patient's version of the medical history) and visuals (the physical findings, nonverbal cues, etc.).

A second way in which reading comics can be valuable in medical education is for their specific thematic relevance. For example, medical educators are concerned with teaching behavioral skills such as empathy, communication, and active listening. Medically themed comics present images and texts that highlight such themes, demonstrating both good and bad examples that provide fodder for discussion. I often introduce a panel from Brian Fies's outstanding comic *Mom's Cancer* (fig. 3.1) to explore the issue of empathy. I show an image of a bald-headed woman with tears streaking down her cheeks and ask students to describe what they see. Inevitably, they identify emotions such as suffering, sadness, pain, and fear, which are clearly expressed by the drawing. This generally provokes further conversation about why she might be feeling these emotions, how doctors ought to respond to their patients' suffering, and ways in which careful observation of body language, nonverbal cues, and context can help students become more empathic and effective clinicians.

Reading comics can also help students practice particular doctoring skills. For example, I use four panels from Marisa Acocella Marchetto's *Cancer Vixen* to discuss the topic of delivering bad news (fig. 3.2). This part of the story takes place soon after the main character, Marisa, visits her physician to evaluate a lump in her breast. The scene begins with Marisa sitting at her drawing table, where the

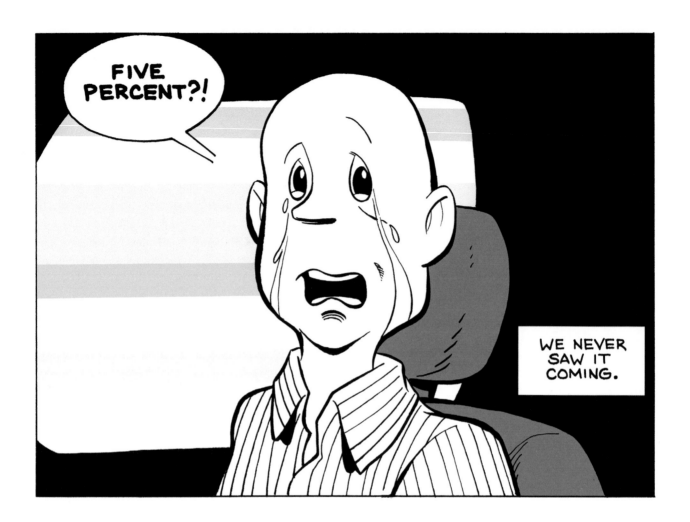

> FIVE PERCENT?!

> WE NEVER SAW IT COMING.

fig. 3.1
From Brian Fies, *Mom's Cancer* (New York: Abrams Image, 2006).

abrupt ringing of a telephone interrupts her. In panel 2, she stands to walk away from the table, literally leaving her familiar world behind as she exits the comic panel. In panel 3, a close-up of the phone shows that Dr. Mills is calling. Then, in the fourth panel, we witness a transformation remarkable for its drama and intensity. A close-up of Marisa's face shows her reaction as Dr. Mills utters nine words on the phone: "Marisa, this is Dr. Mills. There is an abnormality." Marisa's hair stands on end; she covers her eyes, her mouth agape with horror. In a narrative box, she recalls the precise time of the phone call: "10:12 A.M. exactly." In another, "My world came to an end."

In these four panels, the power and impact of the doctor's spoken word is demonstrated clearly and dramatically, showcasing the power of the comics medium for communicating complex emotions and events. The emphasis on the patient's point of view is shown by the use of a close-up of Marisa's phone and her

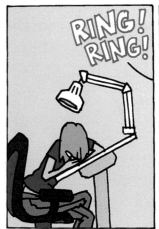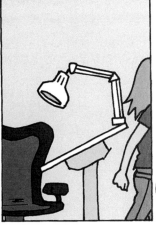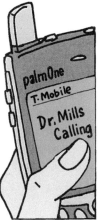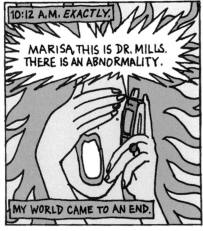

dramatic facial expression as she hears from Dr. Mills. The pacing of the panels shows how these events unfold, demonstrating that the mundane can transform into the indelible in "the blink of an eye." The comic helps students experience at a visceral level the feeling of being on the receiving end of what is likely a routine conversation from the doctor's point of view. Like those with memories of the events of 9/11 or the day JFK was shot, Marisa recalls the exact moment of the phone call. Students often express surprise at the power that doctors' words have to change people's lives in both positive and negative ways, and this stimulates a thoughtful discussion about how physicians should deliver bad news in a sensitive, yet forthright, manner.

The rich and growing corpus of medically themed comics has prompted many related classroom discussions, including:

- The value of observing nonverbal cues
- The importance of attending to the patient's concerns
- Differences between the patient's and the physician's experiences of illness
- The importance of truth telling in medicine
- The role of social and political factors in shaping illness
- The challenges of coping with mental illness and the ambivalence patients may feel about treatment
- The complexity of doctor-patient communication and the implications for informed decision making

Though class readings are varied (ranging from book-length graphic novels to one-page short stories), they share a common focus on illness and/or the medical profession, and they showcase the unique way in which comics can communicate topics with thematic relevance to medical students while also teaching observational and other critical skills necessary for effective doctoring.

Making Comics

In conjunction with reading comics, students enrolled in the course also create their own original comics. This is perhaps the most provocative innovation for a medical school curriculum, and having the students create comics offers several benefits. First, it provides an opportunity for creative expression. Medical school can be a mind-numbingly fallow environment, and students' creativity is systematically squelched at the expense of other curricular goals. Traditional medical school pedagogy ascribes to the "empty vessel" theory of learning, a notion that students' brains merely need to be filled with information provided exclusively by their teachers.[11] This model presumes (incorrectly) that students possess no relevant preexisting competencies other than a willingness and ability to learn. In reality, many medical students have extraordinary and varied talents, which they can rarely express. One goal of the course, then, is to allow students to express themselves creatively around a meaningful medical school experience.

A related goal is to help students improve their communication skills. Students are tasked with telling a compelling story from medical school, using the comic format as a vehicle for communication. By the time students enroll in the course, in their fourth and final year of medical school, they have accumulated experiences and stories with intense personal and professional significance. To transform these stories into comics, students must focus on how to articulate the salient points and lessons clearly, a process that compels them to make decisions and live with the consequences. While the overt task is for students to tell a meaningful story using pictures and words, the blank pages force them to make (and commit to) choices about how to tell the story, who is telling the story, when it takes place, why it unfolds as it does, what is and is not said, how to represent oneself, how to represent others, how to pace the story, and so on. Not only does this teach the importance of point of view, context, and the like, but it also sensitizes students to the relevance of their decisions when communicating in the medical context. The goal is to help students communicate more clearly and concisely, skills that are crucial in healthcare.

Of course creating comics presents medical students with a serious challenge. As individuals accustomed to scholastic success at every level, they are typically confident (which is good) or even arrogant (which is not). Being challenged to tell a story by drawing pictures can be an uncomfortable and often daunting exercise. This humbling lesson is a reminder that they (and doctors in general) seldom have all the answers or skills to solve every formidable problem that comes before them. Nevertheless, by providing a safe setting, an encouraging environment, and the time and opportunity to succeed, students ultimately find satisfaction in their accomplishments, surprise themselves with their abilities, and develop an appreciation for the variety of skills that others might possess in greater quantity.

Finally, making comics is an effective way to facilitate team learning through group interaction. Medicine is a team sport, and I inform students that their course grade depends not only on their individual productivity but also on their willingness and ability to help colleagues create their best work. Thus I require and demand that students help one another as they struggle to express their stories visually. Peer-to-peer feedback helps students build camaraderie and helps them recognize that they will often need assistance to achieve important goals and that they may not know who has the most relevant skill set without looking and asking for help. Despite its intuitive importance, this lesson is typically not taught in the formal curriculum, but it is relevant for life on the wards, where no single person has all the experience, knowledge, and expertise to care for a patient with a complex set of medical, social, and psychological problems.

Since I began teaching this course, students have addressed a variety of issues in their comics, ranging from accounts of personal transformation en route to becoming a doctor to challenges in caring for "difficult" patients. In 2012, Tim Elliott and Brandon Strubberg, then graduate students in English at Texas Tech University, conducted a rhetorical analysis of the themes found in four years of these comics, focusing their attention on the depiction of the students' interactions with both physicians and patients. Of the 153 student-physician interactions they identified, only 19 percent were assessed as "positive" interactions, with 35 percent considered "negative" and 46 percent "neutral." Of the 45 interactions between healthcare professionals and patients, 44 percent were found to be "empathic," 7 percent "non-empathic," and 49 percent "neutral."[12] While these proportions may not reflect the real-world incidence of particular interactions involving medical students, the analysis does provide a glimpse into students' lived experiences. Even if the negative intraprofessional interactions are uncommon, they are nevertheless sufficiently memorable that students feel compelled to retell their experiences graphically.

The Taming of Tina

Several panels from one student's comic illustrate some of these very points. This wonderful story, called *The Taming of Tina*, was conceived by Taylor Olmstead, a talented former student who subsequently trained in pediatrics. This story is told from the student's point of view, and it explores the challenges associated with caring for a belligerent young girl who alienates every healthcare professional she encounters. Using self-deprecating humor, Taylor explores how well-intentioned

THE TAMING OF TINA

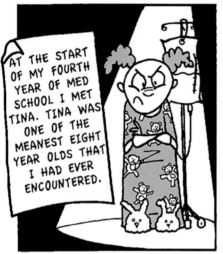

AT THE START OF MY FOURTH YEAR OF MED SCHOOL I MET TINA. TINA WAS ONE OF THE MEANEST EIGHT YEAR OLDS THAT I HAD EVER ENCOUNTERED.

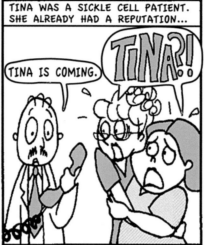

TINA WAS A SICKLE CELL PATIENT. SHE ALREADY HAD A REPUTATION...

TINA IS COMING.

TINA?!

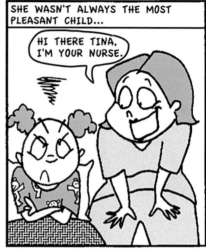

SHE WASN'T ALWAYS THE MOST PLEASANT CHILD...

HI THERE TINA, I'M YOUR NURSE.

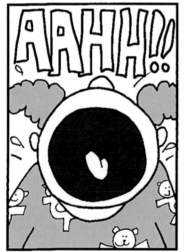

AAHH!!

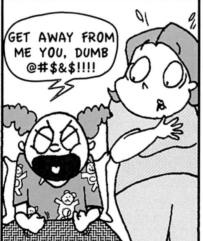

GET AWAY FROM ME YOU, DUMB @#$&$!!!!

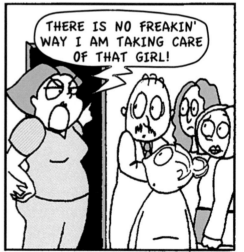

THERE IS NO FREAKIN' WAY I AM TAKING CARE OF THAT GIRL!

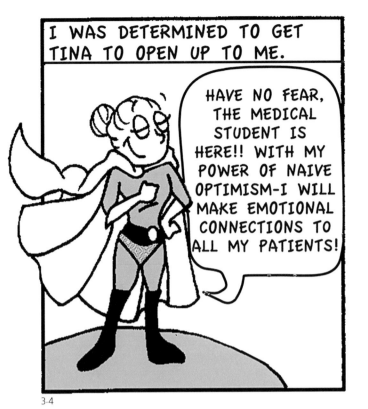

3.4

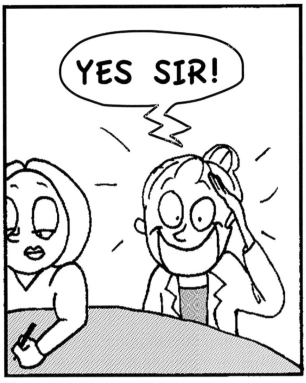

3.5

figs. 3.3–3.5
From Taylor Olmstead, *The Taming of Tina*, 2012.

health professionals often fail to recognize root causes of patients' disruptive behavior and, in doing so, miss opportunities for therapeutic healing.

The opening panels (fig. 3.3) show how Tina terrorizes the entire healthcare team. The patient is depicted in an unsympathetic light, as a foul-mouthed obnoxious girl. The nurses, typically the paragon of compassion, refuse to take care of her, not wanting to be subjected to her serial abuse. The healthcare team's facial expressions show a combination of shock and fear in this surreal scene—a far cry from the typical emotions elicited by sick children.

The author, lacking prior interactions with Tina, at first portrays herself as a superhero (fig. 3.4)—where no one else has succeeded, Taylor will come to the rescue and save the day! But as the story progresses, Taylor evolves, and her character takes on new dimensions that reflect her growing awareness of her role in the medical culture. The superhero soon becomes a naïve novice, keen to please her attending physician and ever hopeful that she will make a difference. This eagerness is humorously demonstrated via the contrast between the wide-eyed grinning student and the weary nurse beside her (fig. 3.5). Next we see Taylor in detective mode, self-assured and determined to get to the bottom of the Tina mystery and ever certain she can be of service (fig. 3.6).

graphic
storytelling and
medical narrative

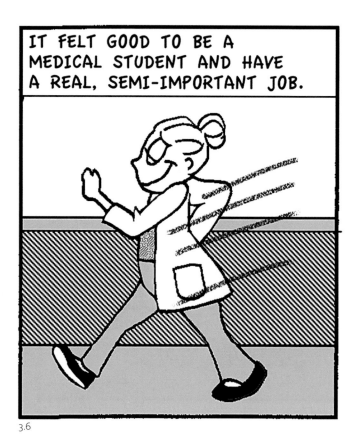

3.6

figs. 3.6–3.8
From Taylor Olmstead,
The Taming of Tina, 2012.

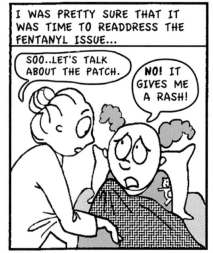

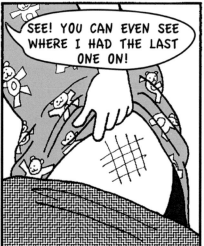

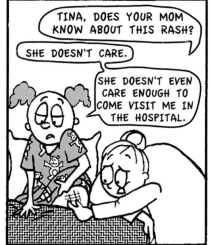

3.7

DID THE MED STUDENT REALLY JUST HUG TINA GOODBYE?
3.8

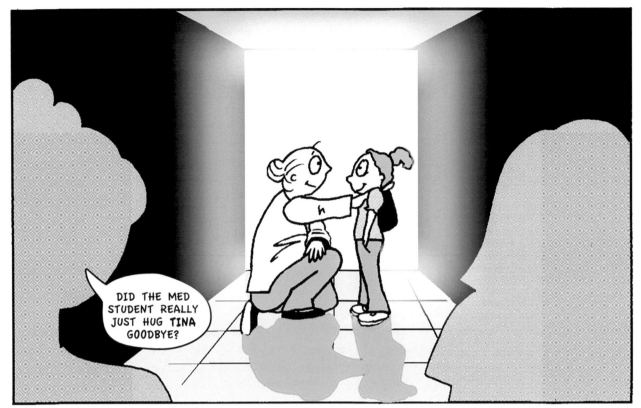

Taylor's enthusiasm is tempered as she encounters numerous barriers to success. When she discovers that the pain patch caused Tina to develop an uncomfortable rash (fig. 3.7), she is rightfully proud of her contribution to the patient's care—though the rest of the medical team seems somewhat less excited by the discovery than Taylor. Nonetheless, through her expressive drawings, we see Taylor integrate her experiences and transform into a more mature and nuanced clinician, still optimistic but realistic as well.

By the close of the story, Taylor assimilates her failures and successes, and she shows herself as an empathic healer—surprising the nurses as she kneels to give Tina a reassuring pat on the shoulder (fig. 3.8). The gesture is tender, and the readers share in Taylor's pride as we come to the realization that she is going to be a terrific doctor.

The story, told with clarity and humor, simultaneously reveals Taylor's personal maturation and mirrors the transformation that all medical students experience on the journey toward becoming physicians. It's touching and funny, and it beautifully demonstrates how the comics medium can be used to express personal as well as professional themes. While this story could doubtless have been told as a traditional textual narrative, the comics medium is ideal for communicating its complex emotions and multiple perspectives. The story's simplicity enhances our understanding of the illness experience and the challenges facing caregivers.

Conclusions

The use of comics in the classroom is not new, but comics have newfound credibility in the medical school curriculum. They can tell compelling stories about illness and demonstrate the complexity of medical culture. Reading comics can help students think critically about the environment in which they learn and work, and making their own comics can help students communicate more clearly and precisely. As comics are further integrated into the curriculum, I look forward to a growing scholarship addressing concrete, measurable outcomes that further demonstrate the unique contributions of comics to medical education.

. . . .

In the following excerpt from Julia Wertz's *The Infinite Wait* (figs. 3.9–3.12), the author brilliantly depicts the complex feelings of uncertainty, frustration, and anger that individuals often experience when trying to make sense of strange symptoms from an undefined illness. Wertz's irritation at the doctors who can't seem to figure out what's wrong with her is eventually transformed into fear and guilt as she learns that the troubling symptoms are explained by a diagnosis of lupus, which, in her mind, might have been self-induced by prescription drug use. For me, the panel that resonates most truthfully is one where Wertz's physician compassionately places a hand on her shoulder and asks how she's feeling. Wertz's response reveals much about the complexity of doctor-patient communication: "Uh-oh, unnecessary touching and terms of endearment? This can't be good . . ."

FIGURES ON
FOLLOWING PAGES

▬ ▬ ▬ ▬ ▬ ▬

figs. 3.9–3.12
From Julia Wertz, *The Infinite Wait and Other Stories* (Toronto: Koyama, 2012).

fig. 3.9

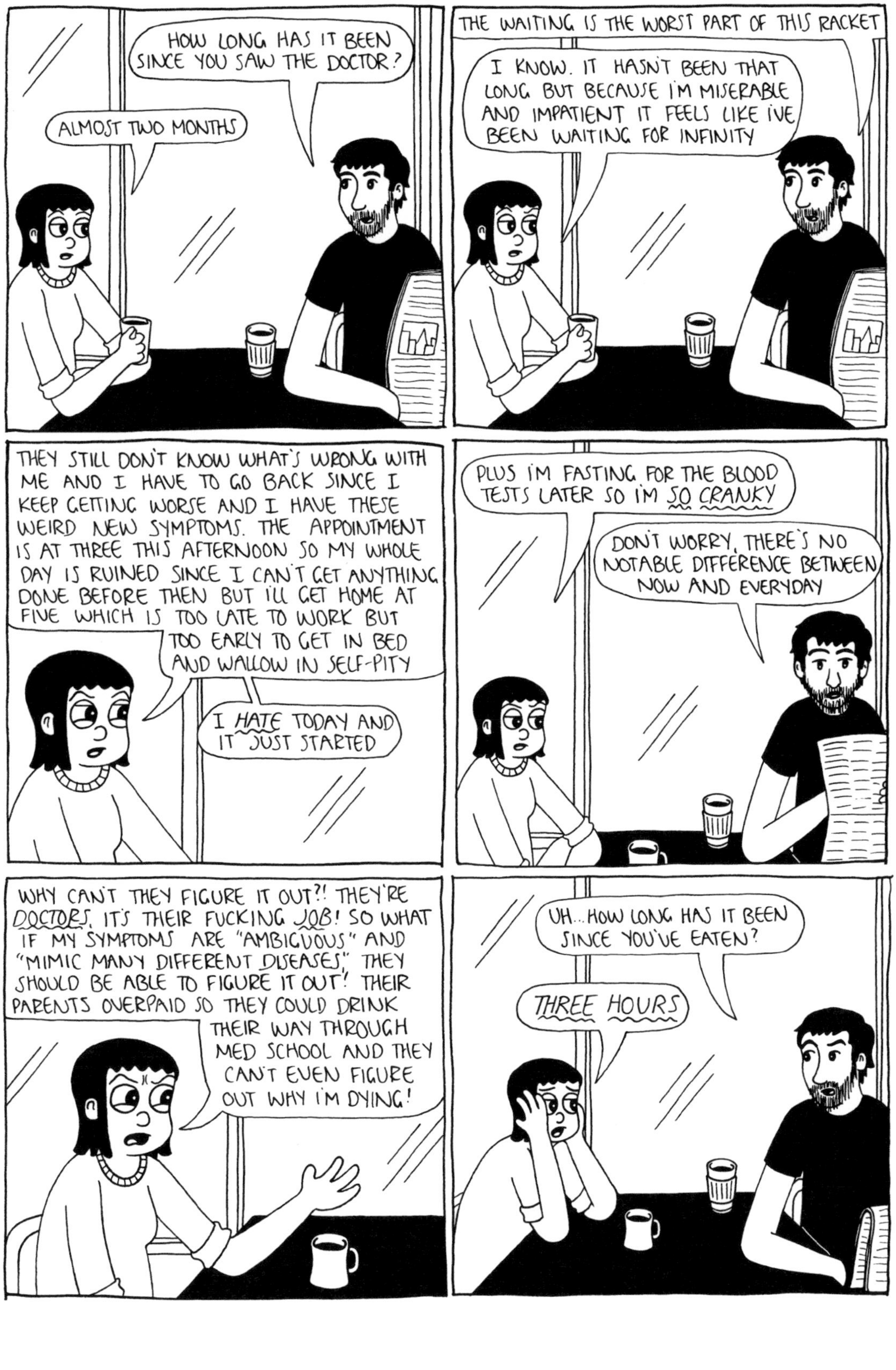
HOW LONG HAS IT BEEN SINCE YOU SAW THE DOCTOR?
ALMOST TWO MONTHS
THE WAITING IS THE WORST PART OF THIS RACKET
I KNOW. IT HASN'T BEEN THAT LONG BUT BECAUSE I'M MISERABLE AND IMPATIENT IT FEELS LIKE I'VE BEEN WAITING FOR INFINITY
THEY STILL DON'T KNOW WHAT'S WRONG WITH ME AND I HAVE TO GO BACK SINCE I KEEP GETTING WORSE AND I HAVE THESE WEIRD NEW SYMPTOMS. THE APPOINTMENT IS AT THREE THIS AFTERNOON SO MY WHOLE DAY IS RUINED SINCE I CAN'T GET ANYTHING DONE BEFORE THEN BUT I'LL GET HOME AT FIVE WHICH IS TOO LATE TO WORK BUT TOO EARLY TO GET IN BED AND WALLOW IN SELF-PITY
I HATE TODAY AND IT JUST STARTED
PLUS I'M FASTING FOR THE BLOOD TESTS LATER SO I'M SO CRANKY
DON'T WORRY, THERE'S NO NOTABLE DIFFERENCE BETWEEN NOW AND EVERYDAY
WHY CAN'T THEY FIGURE IT OUT?! THEY'RE DOCTORS. IT'S THEIR FUCKING JOB! SO WHAT IF MY SYMPTOMS ARE "AMBIGUOUS" AND "MIMIC MANY DIFFERENT DISEASES," THEY SHOULD BE ABLE TO FIGURE IT OUT! THEIR PARENTS OVERPAID SO THEY COULD DRINK THEIR WAY THROUGH MED SCHOOL AND THEY CAN'T EVEN FIGURE OUT WHY I'M DYING!
UH...HOW LONG HAS IT BEEN SINCE YOU'VE EATEN?
THREE HOURS

fig. 3.10

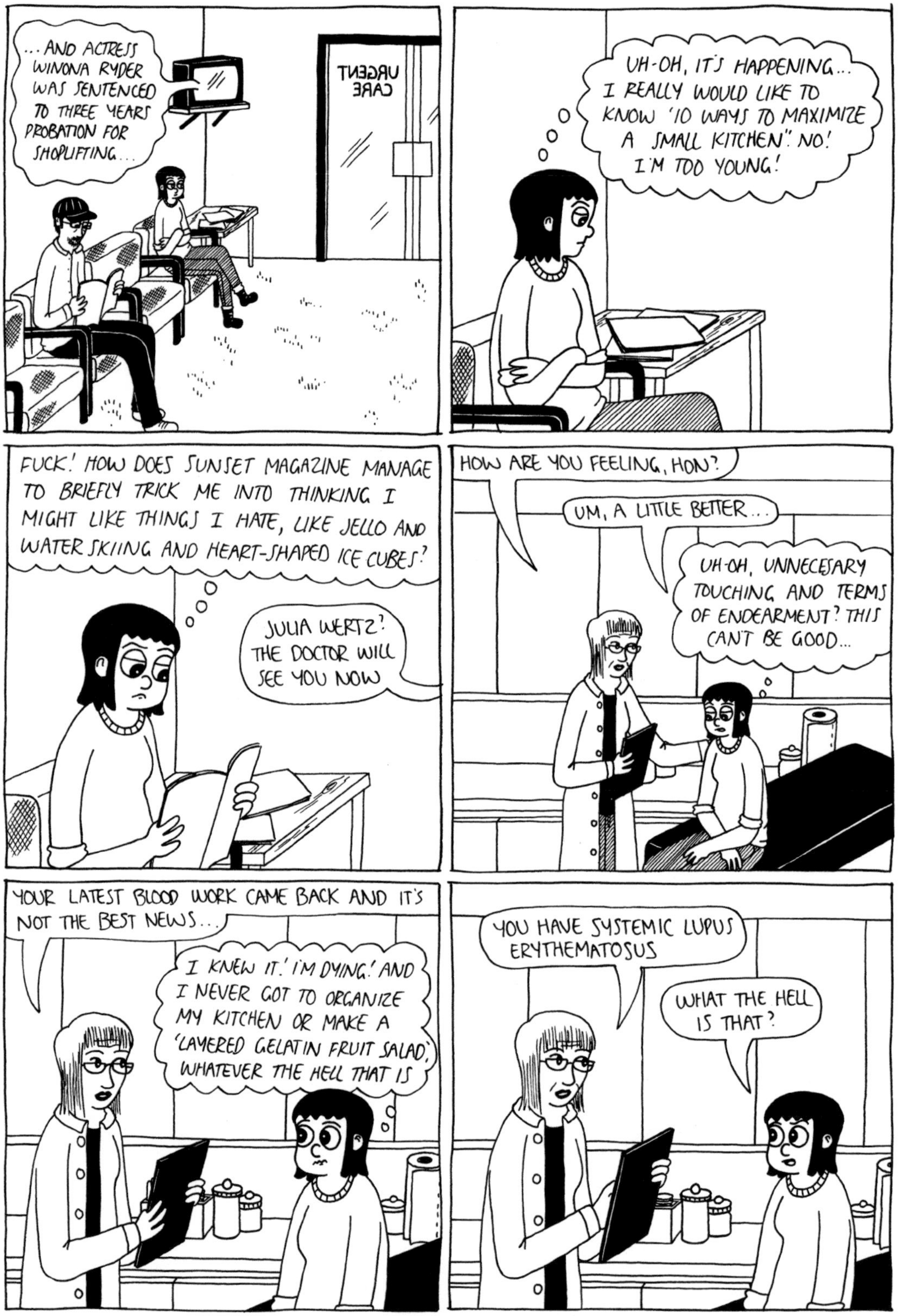
...AND ACTRESS WINONA RYDER WAS SENTENCED TO THREE YEARS PROBATION FOR SHOPLIFTING...
URGENT CARE
UH-OH, IT'S HAPPENING... I REALLY WOULD LIKE TO KNOW '10 WAYS TO MAXIMIZE A SMALL KITCHEN". NO! I'M TOO YOUNG!
FUCK! HOW DOES SUNSET MAGAZINE MANAGE TO BRIEFLY TRICK ME INTO THINKING I MIGHT LIKE THINGS I HATE, LIKE JELLO AND WATER SKIING AND HEART-SHAPED ICE CUBES?
JULIA WERTZ? THE DOCTOR WILL SEE YOU NOW
HOW ARE YOU FEELING, HON?
UM, A LITTLE BETTER...
UH-OH, UNNECESARY TOUCHING AND TERMS OF ENDEARMENT? THIS CAN'T BE GOOD...
YOUR LATEST BLOOD WORK CAME BACK AND IT'S NOT THE BEST NEWS...
I KNEW IT! I'M DYING! AND I NEVER GOT TO ORGANIZE MY KITCHEN OR MAKE A 'LAYERED GELATIN FRUIT SALAD', WHATEVER THE HELL THAT IS
YOU HAVE SYSTEMIC LUPUS ERYTHEMATOSUS
WHAT THE HELL IS THAT?

fig. 3.11

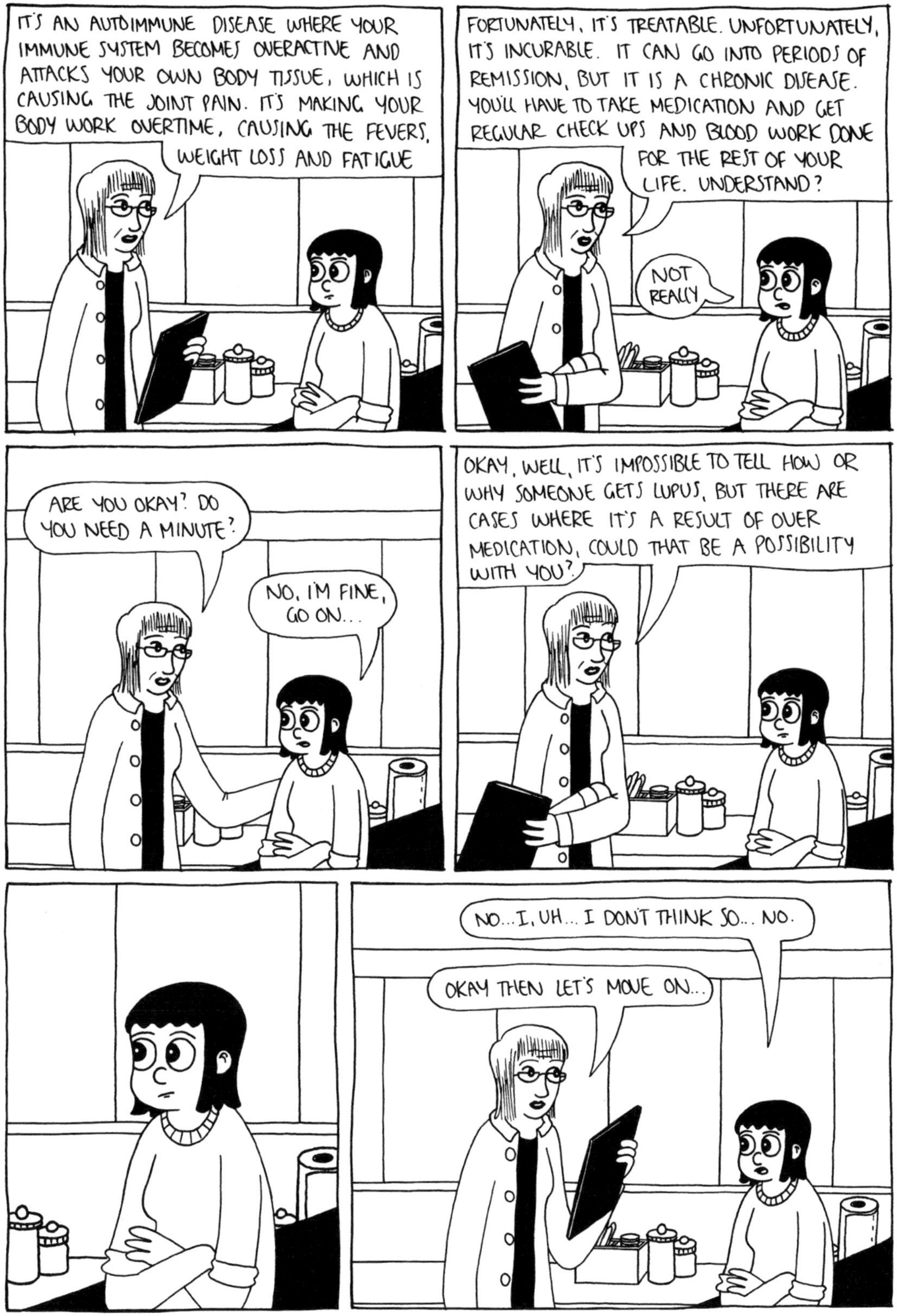
IT'S AN AUTOIMMUNE DISEASE WHERE YOUR IMMUNE SYSTEM BECOMES OVERACTIVE AND ATTACKS YOUR OWN BODY TISSUE, WHICH IS CAUSING THE JOINT PAIN. IT'S MAKING YOUR BODY WORK OVERTIME, CAUSING THE FEVERS,
WEIGHT LOSS AND FATIGUE
FORTUNATELY, IT'S TREATABLE. UNFORTUNATELY, IT'S INCURABLE. IT CAN GO INTO PERIODS OF REMISSION, BUT IT IS A CHRONIC DISEASE. YOU'LL HAVE TO TAKE MEDICATION AND GET REGULAR CHECK UPS AND BLOOD WORK DONE
FOR THE REST OF YOUR LIFE. UNDERSTAND?
NOT REALLY
ARE YOU OKAY? DO YOU NEED A MINUTE?
NO, I'M FINE, GO ON...
OKAY, WELL, IT'S IMPOSSIBLE TO TELL HOW OR WHY SOMEONE GETS LUPUS, BUT THERE ARE CASES WHERE IT'S A RESULT OF OVER MEDICATION, COULD THAT BE A POSSIBILITY WITH YOU?
NO... I, UH... I DON'T THINK SO... NO.
OKAY THEN LET'S MOVE ON...

fig. 3.12

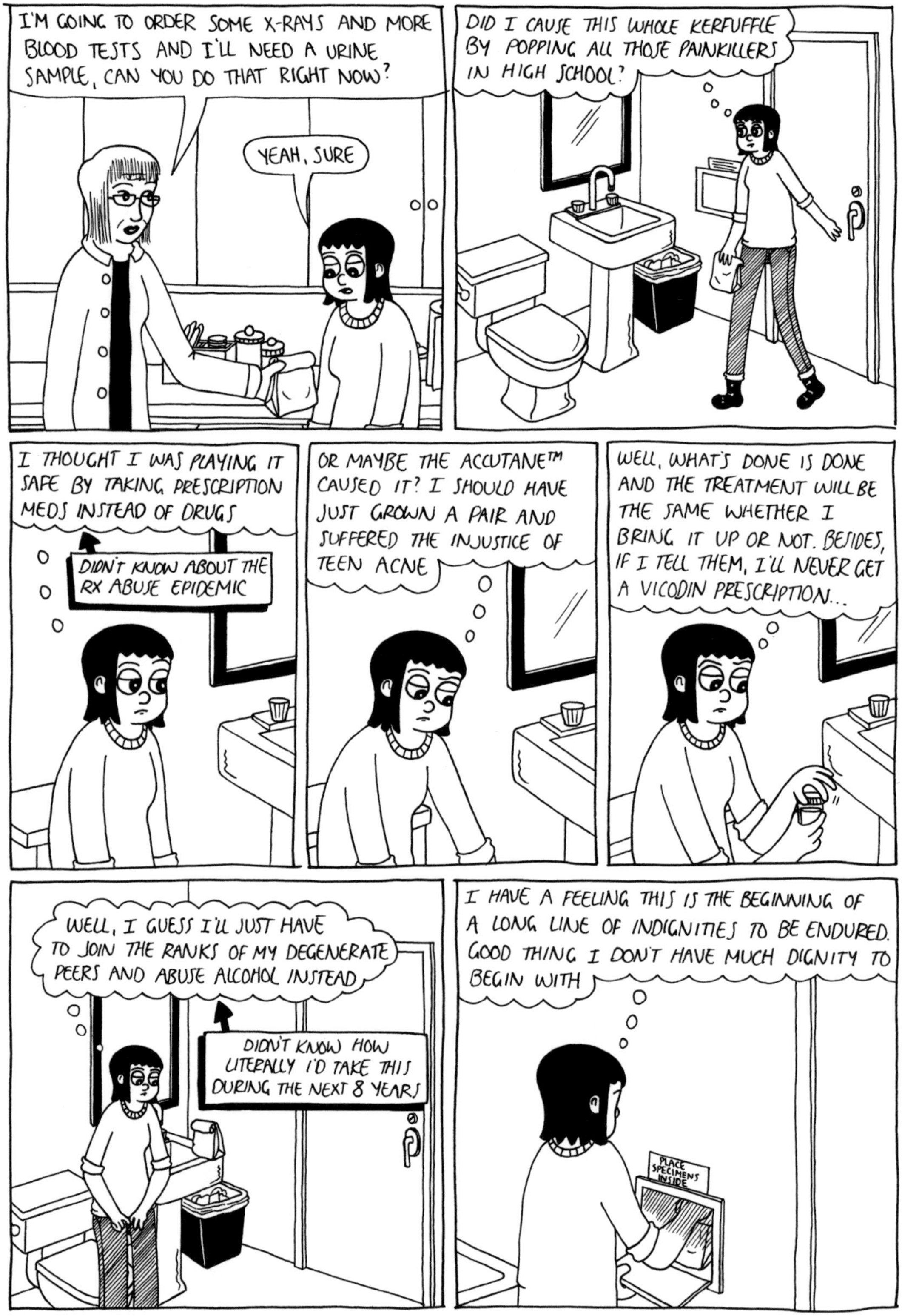
I'M GOING TO ORDER SOME X-RAYS AND MORE BLOOD TESTS AND I'LL NEED A URINE SAMPLE, CAN YOU DO THAT RIGHT NOW?
YEAH, SURE
DID I CAUSE THIS WHOLE KERFUFFLE BY POPPING ALL THOSE PAINKILLERS IN HIGH SCHOOL?
I THOUGHT I WAS PLAYING IT SAFE BY TAKING PRESCRIPTION MEDS INSTEAD OF DRUGS
DIDN'T KNOW ABOUT THE RX ABUSE EPIDEMIC
OR MAYBE THE ACCUTANE™ CAUSED IT? I SHOULD HAVE JUST GROWN A PAIR AND SUFFERED THE INJUSTICE OF TEEN ACNE
WELL, WHAT'S DONE IS DONE AND THE TREATMENT WILL BE THE SAME WHETHER I BRING IT UP OR NOT. BESIDES, IF I TELL THEM, I'LL NEVER GET A VICODIN PRESCRIPTION...
WELL, I GUESS I'LL JUST HAVE TO JOIN THE RANKS OF MY DEGENERATE PEERS AND ABUSE ALCOHOL INSTEAD
DIDN'T KNOW HOW LITERALLY I'D TAKE THIS DURING THE NEXT 8 YEARS
I HAVE A FEELING THIS IS THE BEGINNING OF A LONG LINE OF INDIGNITIES TO BE ENDURED. GOOD THING I DON'T HAVE MUCH DIGNITY TO BEGIN WITH
PLACE SPECIMENS INSIDE

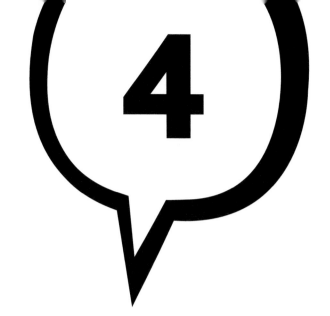

Graphic Pathography in the Classroom and the Clinic

A Case Study

- - - - -

KIMBERLY R. MYERS

Unlike my colleagues, I wasn't a comics junkie growing up. I took myself—my thoughts and my passions—far too seriously and craved what I perceived to be the more nuanced characters of "proper" fiction and biography. I was a ravenous reader as a child, and comics were usually reserved for dessert: I read them as light fare to polish off what sustained me.

But as an adult, I began to look at comics with a more critical eye—*Maus* was the first to captivate me—and realized what my younger, elitist self, for all her good intentions, had missed.[1] Here was a range of comics with characters more psychologically nuanced than the archetypes of good versus evil I had earlier associated with comics, and I began to delight in the clever interplay of word and image. Intrigued by the rise of what we might now call "graphic culture," I was hooked by this medium, which combines intellectual, creative, and psychological sophistication. My formal study of comics came with the advent of graphic pathographies; they were a good fit for my newfound professional focus on literature and medicine.

A few years ago I moved from a department of literature in a university to a department of medical humanities in a college of medicine. Trained as a literary scholar of the romantic, Victorian, and modern periods, my professional foci had, over the course of fifteen years, begun to shift after I was diagnosed with a serious chronic illness. I had slowly branched out, teaching medical humanities for the medical school on our university campus. While I found this hybrid identity—literature professor by day, medical humanities professor by night—satisfying,

The Patient in me wanted to work more fully from within the culture of medicine as a way to make a practical, tangible impact on future physicians, who would then "pay it forward" to their own patients in the form of compassionate care. In a medical school, I reasoned, I would have greater opportunities to enact medical humanities for the good of these two constituencies: healthcare professionals and patients. I currently teach and mentor medical students, and I host a Physician Writers Group for practicing clinicians and soon-to-be residents, helping physicians—current and future—cultivate empathy, good communication skills, and creativity. I also strive to educate patients about medical culture and thereby empower them with some skills to navigate it. I do this in part through my editorship of a medical-center-based literary and visual arts journal as well as through various community outreach projects, including working ad hoc with women who have been diagnosed with breast cancer. Operating from both sides of the divide, I hope to narrow the gap between healthcare professionals and patients. And comics are a useful, engaging way to further this agenda.

This essay contains two distinct sections. The first is an examination of artistic media customarily used in medical education—visual art, photography, and literature—in order to highlight the distinctions of comics as a hybrid medium. The second is a first-person account of how one comic, *Cancer Vixen*, bridged the divide between professional and personal in multifaceted ways within the context of a fourth-year medical course on illness narratives.[2]

Part 1: Aesthetics in Medical Education

Comics are relative newcomers to the aesthetic component of medical education. For decades now, formal courses and one-time events loosely grouped under the heading of "medical humanities" have invited medical students to study literature and visual art as a way to (1) cultivate an understanding of and empathy for patients' experiences with illness, and (2) hone the observational and analytical skills necessary for the successful practice of clinical medicine. Indeed, our program at Penn State College of Medicine utilizes traditional visual "texts" from the very first week of medical education. To illustrate how art can function—and to anticipate how comics can function—as a pedagogical tool in medicine, I invite you to sit in on part of a lecture-discussion, called The Cadaver Experience, that I offer each year to incoming first-year students, students who are understandably anxious about their upcoming course in human anatomy.

I begin The Cadaver Experience with a slide of Rembrandt's *The Anatomy Lesson of Dr. Nicolaes Tulp* as a vehicle to explore some common responses to working with dead bodies. In the painting, an illuminated cadaver lies at the lower center, and a prosector, standing to the right of the cadaver, grips the exposed arm muscles with forceps while lecturing to several anatomists, above and to the left of the cadaver. My students readily notice the conspicuous differences between the seventeenth-century Dutch anatomy experience and their own: the anatomists in the painting are all male and not very young, their dress indicates high social standing, and they aren't actually dissecting the cadaver themselves, only watching as the prosector does so. (Many students also comment on the strange perspective of the cadaver's dissected arm.) The facial expressions and body language of the anatomists, though, are what most interest students, even though they rarely notice these particulars until I prompt them with direct questions.

Here we have a microcosm of the psychodynamics at play in what might be any human anatomy lab. There are "gunners" (i.e., students eager to excel and impress) hovering over the corpse; one is learning all he can by looking at the body, while the other fervently seeks wisdom from his instructor. An anatomist near the prosector gazes across the room quite urgently with an expression something like terror, and another stares into space, head turned and eyes averted from the corpse, which is just beneath him. The anatomist at the apex of the painting looks a little green around the gills, as if he might be sick (a comics artist might use more green than Rembrandt does!). My favorite is the anatomist crouched just behind the gunners, peering over them but protected from close contact with the cadaver by the living bodies of his colleagues. Guiding students to notice subtle details and think about what they might mean serves the new matriculates well during their first week. Most immediately, it alerts them to the fact that people have very different responses to gross anatomy, a formative rite of passage into medical culture, and that no response is "bad." This exercise also sets the stage for the degree of observation and analysis they will be expected to practice, especially during their clinical years.

Although visual art is, in this way, a multivalent genre, literature is sometimes able to conjure images that no paintbrush could, simply because the human imagination is so suggestive and expansive. As the literature scholar in the humanities department of the College of Medicine, I regularly ask students to go beyond merely identifying the issues raised in a literary work in order to explore the subtle implications of how and why the author chooses a certain point of view, style, tone, and the like. A good example is Stephen Crane's novella "The Monster." The crux of this story lies in the ethical tensions between beneficence and nonmaleficence—that is, the obligation to do good and the obligation to do no harm. Even though this ethical dilemma is played out via the badly burned body of Henry Johnson, "the negro who cared for the doctor's horses," Crane does not describe the physical wounds in great detail.[3] Crane does, however, spend considerable time creating extended allusions to the biblical Garden of Eden and the novel *Frankenstein* in order to remind readers of other contexts in which to view this scenario, contexts in which medico-scientific hubris exacts a high price.[4]

As with the Rembrandt painting, students respond well to specific prompts, but they often don't perceive literary subtleties on their own. Perhaps they find art and literature daunting subjects for analysis because they've been led to believe that there's a right way to interpret these forms of "high art"—and that they don't hold the key to unlock those right answers.

Aesthetics and Pathographies

In 2012 I created a course called Pathography: Reading and Writing the Patient, with the goal of providing an opportunity for fourth-year students to return to what brought most of them into medicine in the first place: people and their experiences with illness. More specifically, the course was designed to sharpen analytical skills and deepen narrative competence by examining how and why patients tell their stories of illness in certain ways, as well as to explore the implications of such narrative constructions for both patient and physician. These goals afforded me wide latitude in terms of the texts I would use with medical students, and I was eager to include some of the graphic pathographies (illness narratives in the form of comics) I had been working with as a scholar. *Cancer Vixen*, by Marisa Acocella Marchetto, was at the top of my list.

For a session on breast cancer, then, I searched for fine art depicting mastectomy and found none with the kind of nuance and richness I wanted for teaching observational skills and analysis. I did find photographs, however. Most were merely medical photography. A search of Google Images yielded several tattoos masking post-mastectomy scars and a few photographs of women who had chosen not to undergo reconstructive surgery. William A. Ewing's brilliant collection, *The Body: Photographs of the Human Form*, provided the perfect photograph: *Beauty Out of Damage*, by Matuschka. I also included breast cancer pathographies of three different genres—a first-person narrative, a sequence of four poems by a single poet, and a transcription of an interview of a patient conducted by her physician—from my book, *Illness in the Academy*. These texts, along with Marchetto's graphic pathography, worked well as a group. On the whole, students responded differently to each genre, and, in turn, each genre enabled students to comprehend a different dimension of the experience of breast cancer.

Artistic Medium and Student Response

Although photography is a form of visual art, students aren't as reticent to venture interpretations of photographs—at least those that seem not to have been self-consciously altered by software—as they are about paintings. Of course, photographers, like other visual artists, make choices about framing, perspective, composition, lighting, contrast, texture, rhythm, balance, and so on. But because the subject seems less mediated—or manipulated—by the photographer, students feel more confident in their observations, as though they're observing ordinary life. (In fact, this perception sometimes becomes an impediment to analysis/discussion, when students don't consider the conscious aesthetic choices of the photographer.) Even with provocative photographs, like the nudes of Robert Mapplethorpe, for instance, students feel justified in having an opinion, perhaps because, after all, it seems that anyone might pick up a camera and shoot a photograph, whereas not everyone can wield a paintbrush. In short, photography seems a more transparent medium.

Beauty Out of Damage startles students when it is first projected on a screen—not so much because of the shocking appearance of Matuschka's scar (fourth-year students are used to such scars) but because of the tensions between private and public, disfigurement and glamour. Nevertheless, because the subject is a real woman, students feel as though they are capable of making valid observations. That is, initially, at least, little artistic gap exists, as it might with a painting whose subject appears less realistic. As the process continues, however, because the woman is real, students realize that they are more comfortable adopting either a strictly medical gaze or viewing the woman clothed—but not both, which would require them to view her in an uncomfortable liminal state between patient-in-clinic and person-they-might-meet-in-a-social-setting. Not surprisingly, they almost invariably choose the former and thus medicalize the body.

When I ask them to notice how lighting creates focus, they realize that the swath of brightness across the woman's chest creates a certain visual field not unlike the surgical field created by draping, which provides a way for the surgeon to focus his or her attention on the site of malignancy in order to perform the necessary operation without distraction. The field of vision in this photograph focuses attention on the juxtaposition that students initially find jarring. Here, the patient is out of context; she doesn't wear a hospital gown or even street clothes, as one would expect a cancer patient to wear. Likewise, her scarf is not merely to cover hair loss; it is dramatic, a "statement scarf." Indeed, this person's hair has already returned—or has not (yet) been lost. Perhaps her surgery occurred before chemotherapy. So what do we do with this tension between wellness and illness? These questions lead students to realize that the woman or the photographer (here both, as this is a self-portrait) is raising questions about self-identity vis-à-vis cultural expectations of people with breast cancer . . . and, by extrapolation, about the cultural expectations of people with any disease that disfigures. Such "close reading" of this visual text helps students realize how symbolic something so realistic can be. The Google Image search results are useful transitions to "Reconstruction," in the *Breast Art* series of poems by Lisa Katz. Like the women in the Google photos, Katz dares the reader-viewer to look at her, full-on.

"Reconstruction"

You say I should rebuild
with a sack of plastic, or
one part of the body
replaces another.

A woman might love
a man without a leg.
They can have children.
And men whose legs
don't work
make children
with women who climb on.
Sometimes a child disappears
like a lost limb.

Couldn't we have
a different aesthetic,
asymmetrical,
Japanese,
because of the war,
because islands get invaded.

Couldn't we
admire the ruined, the torn, the perfect
error, because the weaver
skips a row
for the sake of humility,
because your love
needs a few stitches?

See the scar,
the flat plain on my chest.
Connect the dots.
You won't get many chances
to look at an absence straight on.

"Reconstruction" is a wonderful complement to the photograph by Matuschka, and students discover additional considerations as they examine the visual and verbal texts in tandem. Katz immediately engages the reader with the initial word "You" and, later, forces the reader's mind's eye to an imagined "flat plain on my chest" with the word "See" that begins the final stanza. While Katz's reader could be anyone, her intended audience seems especially likely to be medical professionals, as they would be the ones urging her to "rebuild / with a sack of plastic" and to imagine resilient others whose loss of a body part only minimally impacts sexuality; medical professionals would also be in a position to "connect the dots," literally the dots drawn on the skin before surgery or, metaphorically, dots that represent the scars following mastectomy. Despite the fact that students are among the targeted audience for this poem, their responses are less spontaneous—likely because the very arrangement of lines on the page signals "poem" and its sequela, "hard to understand." Moreover, in general, medical students tend to prefer the literal—or what appears to be literal—to the metaphorical, the empirical to the theoretical, the quantitative to the qualitative, perhaps especially after three years of training that privileges such approaches. Because of these preferences—and the training that has convinced them that they must arrive at a single right answer—medical students are daunted by the rhetorical gaps in this poem, its lack of connective tissue that would guide them to a more solid understanding of the poet's "point." ("What's the connection between a child's disappearance and a lost limb?" "What do wars and islands have to do with reconstructive surgery?" "Who's the weaver here, and what does humility have to do with anything?")

Therefore, in this poem, students focus on the more straightforward first and last stanzas in order to debate the benefits and burdens of reconstructive surgery. Also, because it is something tangible that they have seen in the operating room, students quickly move into more familiar discussions of how and when to mark patients prior to surgery, thereby slighting what others might consider the more nuanced considerations of the poem—such as cultural and aesthetic norming, the utility and casualties of metaphorizing disease, and the concepts of "picturesque" and "wabi-sabi" from the domain of visual art. These require prompting. Not so with comics, though.

Part 2: *Cancer Vixen* in the Classroom

Cancer Vixen was not only the most successful text for this session, but it was also the most successful text for the entire course.[5] I believe this is true for two reasons. First, as a comic, it is assumed to be accessible. Students associate comics with their youth—when reading was simply a diversion, a pleasure in its own right—and with contemporary culture, an increasingly icon[o]graphic culture in which text and image work synergistically. Having cut their teeth on Mac computers and smartphones, most students move and learn with ease in this culture, and, consequently, in this medium of graphic pathography. They like it. It is familiar. It is fun. Second, Marchetto's comic is so richly textured that students delight in peeling back the layers of meaning, toggling between image and text, and considering them jointly in order to arrive at multiple understandings. For some reason, students seem not to expect a single correct interpretation. Instead, they are more

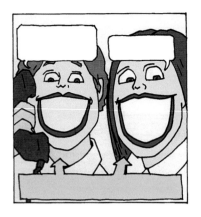

fig. 4.1
From Marisa Acocella Marchetto, *Cancer Vixen: A True Story* (New York: Alfred A. Knopf, 2006). Modified by the author.

playful with the text, open to its possibilities. In order to focus not only on the ideas Marchetto addresses but also on her methods, I alter some individual panels before projecting them in order to slow down Marchetto's process and enable students to see how the parts work together.

As soon-to-be interns (who will be in charge of patients for the first time), fourth-year students are anxious about what it means to be a professional. Reading pathographies, they are as fully interested in depictions of physicians as they are interested in depictions of patients. In short, they are reading/viewing to understand themselves as much as they read/view to understand patients. With this in mind, I choose a single panel and strip the text boxes, leaving only the image of the two (presumed) nurses with hyper-wide smiles and hyper-open eyes (*Cancer Vixen*, 2; fig. 4.1).

Students pounce on the fact that white coats are present, and this detail propels them into speculation. I have questions to guide them into more nuanced observation in case they get sidetracked:

- "How do we 'read' these smiles?"
- "Do the eyes affect your interpretation of the smiles?"
- "Mimic these expressions. Does this give you a visceral clue to what these white-coats are experiencing?"
- "Have you ever smiled this way? If so, in what context?"
- "What do these facial expressions indicate?"

After we discuss these things, I project another slide, showing the panel to the left of the first one (fig. 4.2). Students now have an even clearer context for their interpretation, seeing the same exaggerated smile on the face of the doctor who stands over an exposed breast without looking at it—and certainly not looking into the face of the patient supine on the table before him. Avoidance, then; trying to cover something uncomfortable, like bad news that has emerged during a physical exam.

When I then insert the upper text boxes for the nurses (fig. 4.3), students speculate on how the dialogue interfaces with the image. That the "doctor will see you in an hour" is a sentinel detail, potentially signaling a sense of urgency. Students have just experienced the perspective of the patient during this exercise—initially unsure what's going on but increasingly uncomfortable that something bad is being covered up. Incrementally, they come to understand what Marchetto did, and this is when I add her take on the experience, as conveyed in the lower text box (2; fig. 4.4).

This analysis of Marchetto's panels invites students to consider how the body language and facial expressions they so carefully cultivate—for all the right reasons—sometimes don't put patients at ease at all. What's more important, the

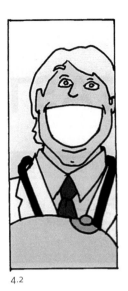

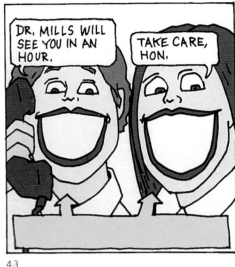

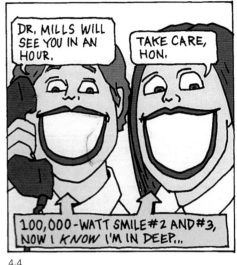

4.2

4.3

4.4

fig. 4.2–4.3
From Marisa Acocella Marchetto, *Cancer Vixen: A True Story* (New York: Alfred A. Knopf, 2006). Modified by the author.

fig. 4.4
From Marisa Acocella Marchetto, *Cancer Vixen: A True Story* (New York: Alfred A. Knopf, 2006).

fig. 4.5
From Marisa Acocella Marchetto, *Cancer Vixen: A True Story* (New York: Alfred A. Knopf, 2006). Modified by the author.

technique of "layering" comics induces students to read more attentively for processes instead of merely reading for issues and plotlines.

Another sequence gives students visceral insight into the degree of anxiety a patient feels when awaiting test results (6). I begin with the first panel, devoid of text boxes, and the final borderless panel (fig. 4.5). Looking at these together, students understand that the cell phone is the patient's sole focus; it is literally the only thing in her range of vision when it rings. That she receives fifty-seven calls indicates a pressing issue of some sort, especially as Marchetto can number the calls from each member of her primary support group: fiancé, best friends, and mother. That Marchetto includes "doctors" in this list indicates the weight of their significance to her in this moment, and the understated "0" Marchetto draws to indicate the number of calls she has received from these doctors depicts a glaring contrast. (Students often talk here about how they would draw the telephone from their perspective and how they would indicate the number and recipients of

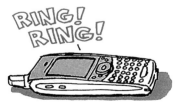

4.5

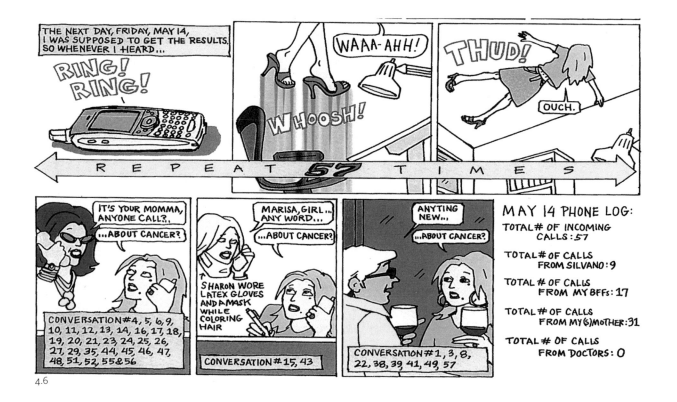

4.6

figs. 4.6–4.8
From Marisa Acocella Marchetto,
Cancer Vixen: A True Story (New York:
Alfred A. Knopf, 2006).

phone calls they make on a single day—casual comments that unexpectedly and fruitfully broaden the discussion.)

While this two-panel excerpt kindles students' understanding of what Marchetto wants to convey, the intervening panels drive home her point (6; fig. 4.6). Every time the phone rings, Marchetto is so startled that she feels as though she is sucked out of her chair into the air with a force that slams her into the ceiling. These calls are all dead ends, false alarms that add to her discomfort ("ouch"); she has no capacity to move beyond the walls (or ceiling) of her room, metaphorically speaking, to become proactive because she does not receive the information she needs to proceed. Again, Marchetto emphasizes this point with the text arrow that spans the first three panels in the sequence: "Repeat 57 Times," the 57 in a bold red font. The grinding tedium of such continually thwarted expectation is underscored by the numbers that crowd the lower text boxes, and her growing exhaustion is evident in her eyes and mouth.

When the dreaded call finally comes, Marchetto registers, in close-up, Dr. Mills's name on the screen of her PDA (7; fig. 4.7). This is the name she has been waiting to see, and it fills the screen as fully as it commands her attention. And then immediately, the next panel conveys the impact of Dr. Mills's report (7; fig. 4.8). By this point, there is no need to analyze the panel part-by-part. Students are

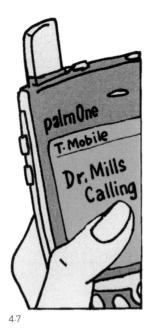

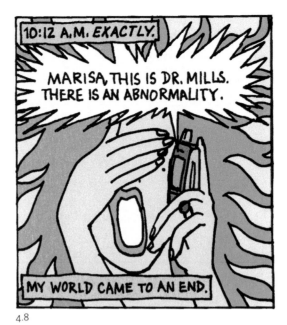

4.7 4.8

attuned to the kinds of lines Marchetto uses to convey bad news: her hair stands straight out and up, and the dialogue bubble is not the typical curvilinear one but rather angular, spiked to indicate the news that will impale her. Her precision in time—"10:12 A.M.," instead of, say, rounding it off to the quarter-hour—and the italicized word "*exactly*" complement the text box at the bottom of the frame: "My world came to an end" (7).

Ironically, so would mine.

Cancer Vixen in the Clinic

Discussing this particular text in such minute detail with my students made me a bit uneasy. My annual mammogram was coming up the next day, and, as any woman might do, I couldn't help placing myself in Marchetto's position, wondering "What if?" The timing of this session on breast cancer seemed especially inauspicious in light of other events that were, I thought, too numerous to be coincidental: my recent presentation on breast cancer pathographies at an international conference, a colleague's recent diagnosis of breast cancer, my sudden and inexplicable affinity for newsboy caps that led me to buy three of them, and the return of a dull ache in my left breast that had waxed and waned over the course of two decades. I was eerily aware of the confluence of these events, and I tried to stave off my deepening sense of foreboding with the rhetorical question, "So what are the odds that you would be diagnosed with breast cancer just when so many vectors in your life right now point toward breast cancer?" Pretty good odds, as it turns out.

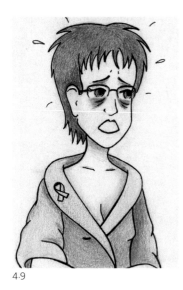

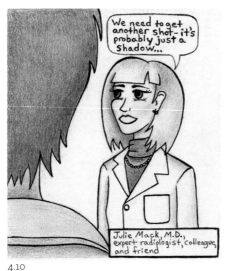

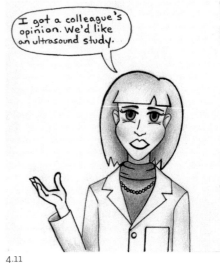

4.9

4.10

4.11

figs. 4.9–4.13
Comic by Pamela Wagar Smith.

Fewer than twenty-four hours after discussing Marchetto's text with my students, I was undergoing many of the procedures—and the emotions—she so memorably depicts in *Cancer Vixen*. I can't be sure if someone who casually reads a comic recalls details as vividly as one who teaches a comic, but Marchetto was my constant companion throughout the entire next day . . . and several of the days in the weeks and months to come. For one thing, while I was waiting in the "diagnostic room" to be called back for my imaging study, I kept thinking about various ways I would draw myself at that moment—if I had had the presence of mind to focus on drawing instead of on the anxiety that was consuming me. It might have looked something like figure 4.9.

While I was waiting for the mammogram, a radiologist colleague and friend of mine, Dr. Julie Mack, saw me and asked if I would like her to read my study. (We have co-authored an essay about this experience from our different perspectives, published in the Winter 2013 issue of *Atrium*.[6]) I had already arranged to wait for the test results and was very pleased that she would be reading the image. When the pictures had been taken, the technician asked me to remain in the exam room while she made sure that Julie had all the shots she needed. I was expecting the technician to return. Instead, Julie came into the room (fig. 4.10).

I knew from past experience that the need for additional images didn't necessarily mean anything bad, but hearing this—especially from the radiologist herself—fanned my fear. When I saw Julie coming down the hall after the second set of pictures had been taken, I could tell immediately that everything was not okay (fig. 4.11).

Following the third set of images, Julie did not return for a very long time. I sat in the diagnostic waiting room, marking each second as it passed. I was keenly

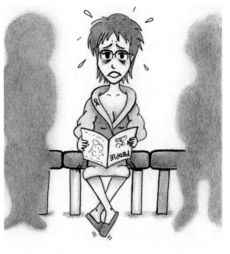

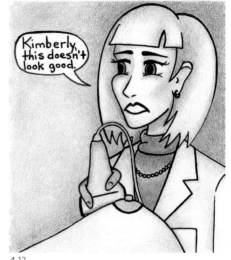

4.12   4.13

aware of how large and bulky the Breast Center robe was on my petite frame, keenly aware of how blank my mind was except for the overwhelming sense of terror
that consumed me, keenly aware that there were two other women waiting in that
room but that the only thing I could do was turn the pages of a magazine without
seeing (much less reading) anything that was on them (fig. 4.12).

In the few flashes of lucidity I had, I kept returning to Marchetto's process,
deciding how I would visualize and verbalize my experience in that moment. The
only similarity between Marchetto's depiction and my own sonogram was the
look of terror on our faces as the probe rolled over our breasts (fig. 4.13). In my
case, the room was quite dim. For a while, I stared at the ceiling, waiting breath-
lessly (literally holding my breath) for Julie to say that everything was okay. She
didn't.

Because she was a friend, Julie was able to move things along all in one sitting so that I didn't have to return multiple times for multiple tests. The returning
wouldn't have been so bad, except that it would have entailed waiting. And waiting for procedures or the results of those procedures is my idea of hell. Just like
Marchetto's panels about The Call.

Next came the core needle biopsy, and this is when Marchetto was most fully
present in my own medical suite. I felt myself morph into the bug-eyed patient in
Marchetto's frame and realized that most of what I was hearing was squiggles (89;
fig. 4.14). That is, I literally couldn't hear—or recognize—the technical language
used by the radiologist and technician; I couldn't make sense of it. I heard only
individual words and phrases as they were performing the needle biopsy. And,
because I was desperate to exchange my patient status for that of colleague—no
doubt to reclaim some semblance of control—I began telling Julie about *Cancer*

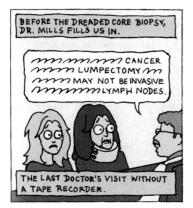

BEFORE THE DREADED CORE BIOPSY, DR. MILLS FILLS US IN.

~~~~~~~ CANCER
~~~~~ LUMPECTOMY ~~
~~~~ MAY NOT BE INVASIVE
~~~~~~~ LYMPH NODES.

THE LAST DOCTOR'S VISIT WITHOUT A TAPE RECORDER.

4.14

figs. 4.14–4.15
From Marisa Acocella Marchetto,
Cancer Vixen: A True Story (New York:
Alfred A. Knopf, 2006).

Vixen. I remember describing this particular panel to her and telling her how the students and I had discussed it. I believe she was glad that I was talking while she was punching out the "biopsied wormy bastards," as Marchetto calls the specimens (89).

A lot transpired on that winter Friday. Although I didn't have pathology results to confirm my diagnosis, both Julie and another friend who specializes in breast surgery for cancer patients left little room for wishful thinking. People's responses to breast cancer are as individual as their cancers themselves and the treatments prescribed for them. I can understand many reasons why women choose not to reveal their diagnoses, but I did not want to hide mine. For one thing, it seemed the perfect teaching/learning moment. In every course I teach, I strive to help students cultivate a real community of trust, openness, and vulnerability; usually, it works. This was an opportunity to practice what I preach.

Taking Marchetto Back to Class

Still mostly numb, I went into class on Monday and carried out the activities we had scheduled, including Skyping with two people whose pathographies we would later read. When these interviews were over, I began, "Remember what we were discussing this time last Thursday? Well, last Friday was my annual mammogram, and. . . ."

I was initially struck by how having read and discussed the breast cancer pathographies made discussing my real-time experience so much easier, which confirmed my longtime suspicion that using pathographies in the clinic would be an excellent tool for doctor-patient communication and patient empowerment. The fourth-year students, soon to be residents, were eager to understand how the experiences conveyed in our texts corresponded to my recent experience. *Cancer Vixen*, in particular, gave them and me excellent points of departure. For instance, Marchetto was not surprised and was seemingly untroubled when her primary care physician asked her about the lump in her breast during an exam (2; fig. 4.15).

I, however, was acutely overwhelmed, to the point I thought I would pass out on the sonogram table. The students and I returned to Marchetto's depiction of the minute her "world came to an end," and they asked me how I would convey my experience (fig. 4.16). In this way, the students and I were essentially co-creating a graphic pathography, where tweaking the details—their asking me "Is this the right color?" and "What would you put here?"—clarified issues that would be important for our continued work that semester and, indeed, for me as well, throughout the year of treatment that lay ahead.

A second example illustrates this point. Marchetto conveys her panic in a four-panel sequence in which water continues to rise (68; fig. 4.17). Students had earlier identified this sequence as one of the most effective in the book, as it

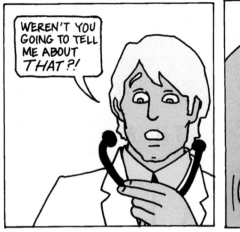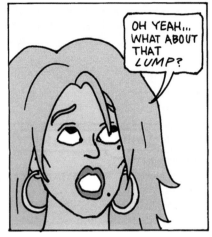

4.15

expertly exploits many of the conventions of the comics medium (e.g., the repetition of the focal image that changes in the fourth panel, the easy integration of the surreal, and the effect of the initial framing caption). The words "salt water fish" indicate that this water is her tears, and her avatar's gasping for breath in the final panel indicates that Marchetto is metaphorically drowning in her fear. Using this sequence as a springboard, the students and I explored how my response differed significantly from Marchetto's. After the biopsy, I shakily dressed and met George, another physician friend of mine, who had come to wait with me for our surgeon friend, who would see me after his clinic ended.[7] I cried briefly when I first saw George. But then I got very still and was numb. I was aware of feeling incoherent as I kept circling back to the basic issue: I had breast cancer. The point was that I needed to talk about it—not call everyone close to me to let them know but just talk until I could get my head around the shock. Unlike Marchetto, I had no outward emotion; my energy was almost entirely cerebral. Neither did I experience Marchetto's anger (69) or her questioning "Why is this happening to me?" (71).

Talking about these contrasts empowered the students as budding clinicians. I was struck by their professionalism and maturity as the power dynamic in the classroom shifted for the day: I was a vulnerable patient who welcomed any medical information they might have, and they were eager to impart that information in case it might assuage my anxiety about what was yet unknown. Because we had discussed how my experience had differed from Marchetto's, they knew some important information about how best to care for me even as they could not cure me.

This experience created a bond between teacher and students unlike anything I had ever experienced. After that day, except for a couple of very brief updates—including confirmation of diagnosis and, later, stage of tumor—our work in the classroom went on in the usual way: I was their professor and they were

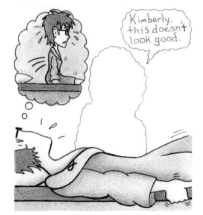

fig. 4.16
Comic by Pamela Wagar Smith.

figs. 4.17–4.18
From Marisa Acocella Marchetto,
Cancer Vixen: A True Story (New York:
Alfred A. Knopf, 2006).

4.17

my students. Marchetto followed me around in my private life, though, providing me a kind of virtual community and, in fact, information that proved to be quite useful.

So many times I saw myself engulfed by the specter of cancer that seemed to run amok around me (83; fig. 4.18). Marchetto doesn't even need to finish the sentence she begins in the upper text box. The drawing makes her message perfectly clear: every aspect of life, no matter how pleasant on the outside, is permeated by thoughts and fears of cancer. Cancer preoccupies; it invades every inch of space. Its often unspoken presence is unchecked, haphazardly proliferating, like the erratic cell division that characterizes the disease itself.

Cancer is a world unto itself, and not even my friends who are physicians had very much to offer me in the way of information about the protocols and procedures specific to oncology. Marchetto did, though. In fact, I am convinced that physicians could use graphic pathographies to empower their patients largely because *Cancer Vixen* helped me in so many concrete ways. I was surprised at just how quickly other people took over when I was diagnosed with breast cancer. Things need to move quickly, and they certainly did for me. Appointments were set up and procedures scheduled; my calendar filled almost instantly. But especially because I was still overwhelmed by this new world I had entered, I needed to slow down so that I could think carefully. I returned to Marchetto to see what—with time and distance, as she was creating *Cancer Vixen*—she had considered important enough to include. I mention only three things to illustrate the utility of this comic in the most serious of circumstances.

First, while I probably would have thought of getting a second opinion, I can't be sure, given how fast things were moving. Marchetto certainly convinced me that having a second opinion is simply a smart thing to do, though, especially when she shows how some things she had been told by one physician were factually incorrect (108–11). I set up an appointment for a second opinion at a leading cancer institute in a nearby city, which helped me understand the range of options available to me.

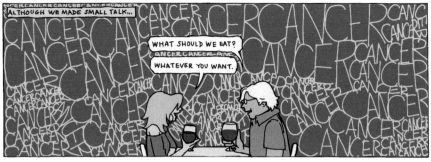

4.18

Second, working in medical humanities, I am well aware of how important it is for patients to have some means of capturing the information their physicians convey to them. I often advise patients to invite a friend to appointments, as two heads have a better chance of remembering details than one, and disagreements over what was said lead to important requests for clarification. I believe it is safe to say that, unless I had read *Cancer Vixen*, I would never have considered taking a digital voice recorder (the equivalent of Marchetto's "tape recorder," 17, 32, 114, 141) to my appointments. Yet that turned out to be absolutely critical as I was trying to decide between two courses of chemotherapy suggested for my particular kind of cancer. I was able to listen to highly technical information as many times as I needed in order to comprehend my options and thereby act with autonomy. On a more basic level, being able to replay fundamental information (about how tumors are typed and staged, in what circumstances chemotherapy is and is not recommended, how oncotypes are determined, and so on) facilitated discussions with family and friends. I returned again and again to listen to what various physicians had explained to me, which helped me feel knowledgeable enough to ask intelligent questions that were crucial to my care.

I chose not to reread *Cancer Vixen* before beginning chemotherapy because I know that every person's experience is unique, and I didn't want to psych myself out by projecting any particular reaction. After completing chemo, however, it was helpful to return to the comic simply to compare Marchetto's experiences with my own. For example, we both experienced the pain of Neulasta injections to boost white cells (164), and we both feared extravasation—which I actually experienced—and subsequent nerve damage (177). However, while Marchetto became preoccupied with gaining weight and losing hair, those concerns seemed utterly inconsequential to me. She continued to work out regularly and maintain a vibrant social life, but I could manage neither. Perhaps the most interesting contrast emerged in our different chemo cocktails and their respective side effects, both long- and short-term: the chemo she had chosen was the one I had rejected. This process provided a powerful sense of community for someone who didn't want to join a support group for fear of collective fearmongering. Ultimately, though only in retrospect, it was helpful to see how my body's terribly unfamiliar responses were actually quite familiar to someone else.

My positive experience with *Cancer Vixen*—both professional and personal—has convinced me that medical comics, in general, and graphic pathographies, in particular, are excellent resources that combine all the best of visual and verbal media. While I remain a strong proponent of using traditional forms of art—painting, photography, literature—to teach medical students, I am especially excited to incorporate more and more graphic medicine into my work with students, physicians, and patients. Indeed, it is our hope that this initial collection of essays will, among other things, inspire graphic artists to create more primary material that will further understanding and interest among healthcare professionals and patients alike.

· · · · · · · · ·

Michael Green and I have illustrated how we use graphic pathographies with our students to help them understand patients' perspectives as they navigate illness. Few comics illustrate how illness affects the other person in the clinic, the healthcare provider—Ian Williams's and MK Czerwiec's cutting-edge work notwithstanding. Fewer still are comics created by medical students attempting to capture, in the moment, their transformation into professionals. We need more work like Ashley Pistorio's *Vita Perseverat* (*Life Goes On*) to fill the void.

Pistorio created this striking ten-page comic when she was a fourth-year medical student in Michael's course, Graphic Medicine and Medical Narratives. In it, Pistorio meets with her neurology attending (i.e., the senior physician, a neurologist, who supervises her). It is late Friday afternoon and, after giving her some constructive criticism on patient notes she has charted, he invites her to "tag along" on late rounds.

Pistorio depicts several themes that recur in discussions among medical students: the need to hide one's emotions—especially fear—from team members, lest one be thought weak and unfit to practice medicine; the conflict between students' individual needs and the needs of their team; a questionable self-image ("I'm just a medical student") freighted with self-doubt (Pistorio's self-infantilization); the chaos not only of physical space filled with cacophonous high-tech machines but also of a universe in which tragic outcomes occur at random; the despair of patients and families; and the isolation, physical and emotional, medical students often experience.

FIGURES ON
FOLLOWING PAGES
▬ ▬ ▬ ▬ ▬ ▬

figs. 4.19–4.28
From Ashley L. Pistorio, *Vita Perseverat*,
2010.

fig. 4.19

VITA PERSEVERAT

By Ashley L. Pistorio

I *began like any other Friday evening. I was on the neurology service, just finishing up late rounds. I stuck around to get some constructive criticism on my patient notes from the attending physician.*

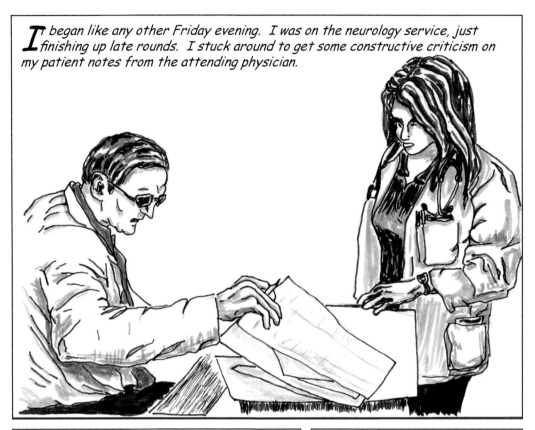

I just have a couple of things to finish up. You're welcome to tag along, or you can go home...

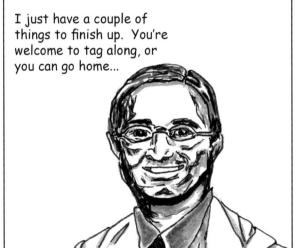

Yeah. Like I actually had a choice.

In medical school, there really is no "optional" clinical activity.

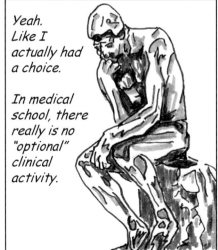

fig. 4.20

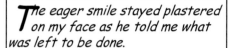

The eager smile stayed plastered on my face as he told me what was left to be done.

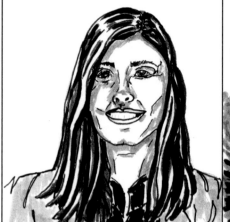

HE HAD TO SEE TWO NEW PATIENTS AND BEGIN THE PROCESS OF DECLARING THEM

BRAIN DEAD

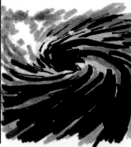

I wanted to run.

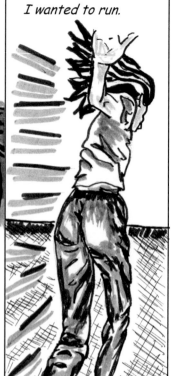

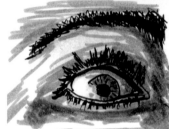

I wanted to hide.

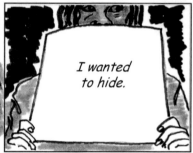

But I had a duty.

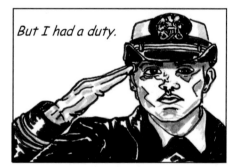

I would have to deal with this one day.

Better now when I'm **just** a medical student. Right?

Okay. Let's go!

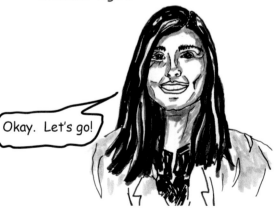

fig. 4.21

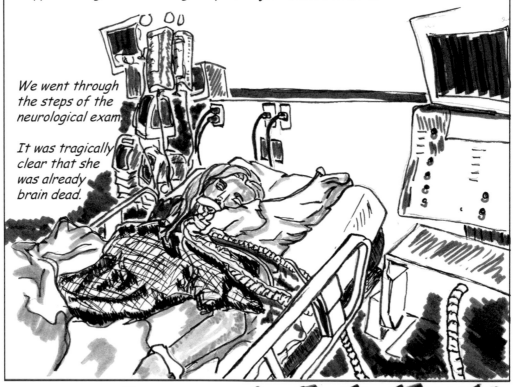

Our first patient was in the medical ICU. She was only 19. She had arrived by helicopter after her grandparents found her unconscious in severe diabetic ketoacidosis. They told us that she started to rebel when she turned 14. She stopped taking her insulin regularly. She just wanted to fit in.

We went through the steps of the neurological exam.

It was tragically clear that she was already brain dead.

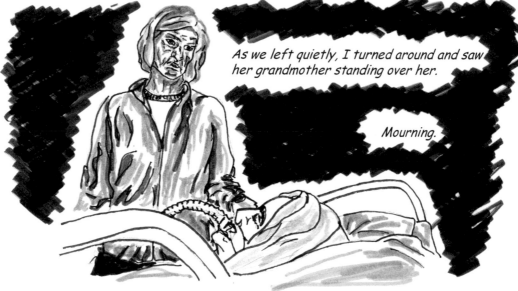

As we left quietly, I turned around and saw her grandmother standing over her.

Mourning.

fig. 4.22

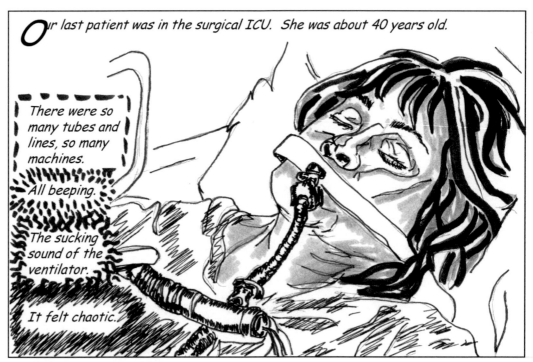

Our last patient was in the surgical ICU. She was about 40 years old.

There were so many tubes and lines, so many machines.

All beeping.

The sucking sound of the ventilator.

It felt chaotic..

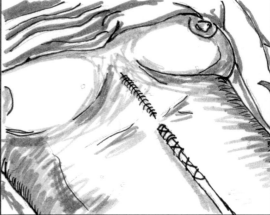

As we performed the exam, I caught bits of her story from the resident that had come in to observe. Early this morning she felt a little short of breath, a slight twinge in her chest. She went to the emergency department at another hospital. They thought she may be having a heart attack, and they wanted to do a cardiac catheterization to try and remove any blockage before there was too much damage.

During the procedure something went horribly wrong. She was rushed to the OR. Now she lay here, in our hospital, lifeless, exposed.

fig. 4.23

Later that night, I struggled to clear the images from my mind...

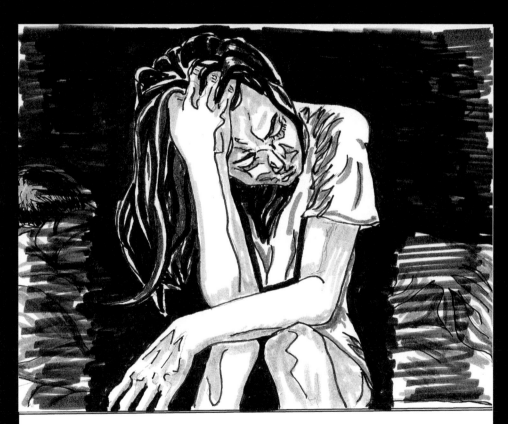

*If I closed my eyes, I saw them. I heard the beeping.
The rhythmic swishing of the ventilator. Cacophony.*

fig. 4.24

On Saturday morning, I reported for patient rounds. We were told by the medical ICU residents that the 19 year old girl had passed away overnight. Her heart finally gave out and her grandparents did not want extraordinary measures. She had already suffered enough.

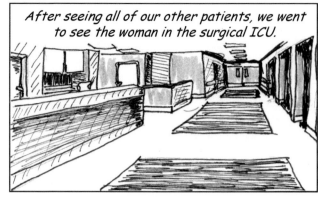

After seeing all of our other patients, we went to see the woman in the surgical ICU.

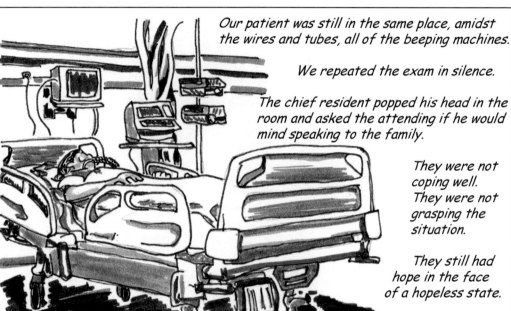

Our patient was still in the same place, amidst the wires and tubes, all of the beeping machines.

We repeated the exam in silence.

The chief resident popped his head in the room and asked the attending if he would mind speaking to the family.

They were not coping well. They were not grasping the situation.

They still had hope in the face of a hopeless state.

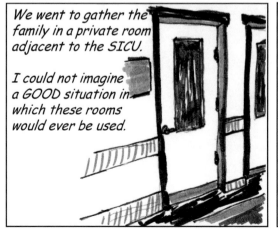

We went to gather the family in a private room adjacent to the SICU.

I could not imagine a GOOD situation in which these rooms would ever be used.

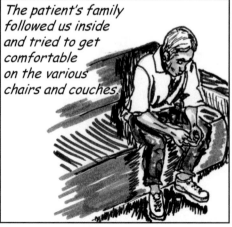

The patient's family followed us inside and tried to get comfortable on the various chairs and couches.

fig. 4.25

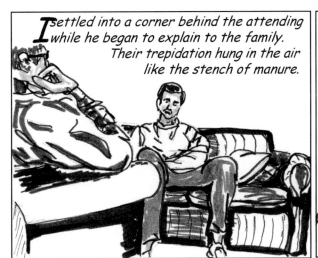

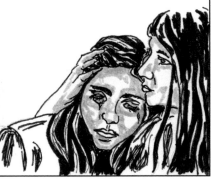

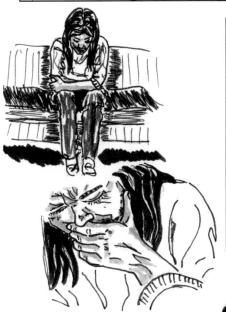

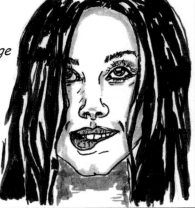

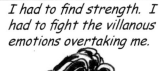

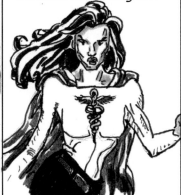

graphic
pathography

fig. 4.26

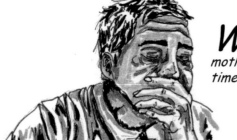

*W*hen his daughter demanded to be allowed to lay in bed with her mother, he broke down for the first time.

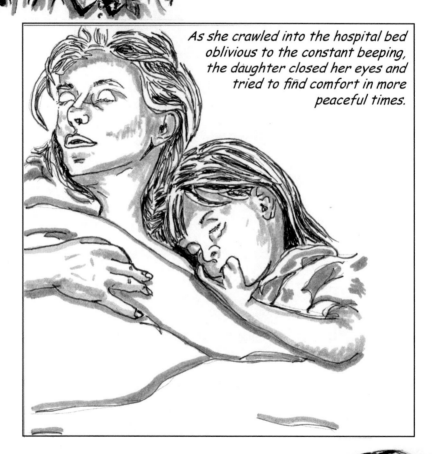

As she crawled into the hospital bed oblivious to the constant beeping, the daughter closed her eyes and tried to find comfort in more peaceful times.

I sat in the work area just outside the patient's room, listening to our group discussing the next steps.

Someone would need to contact the Gift of Life people.

Has anyone called pastoral care? The social worker?

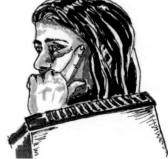

fig. 4.27

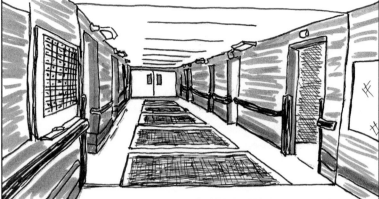

After all of the business of the living dead was finished, we left the SICU. The hallway seemed impossibly long. I excused myself and headed for the only private place I could think of.

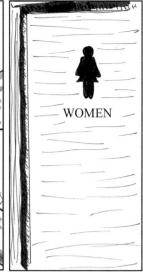

WOMEN

The loss I had witnessed finally overcame me.

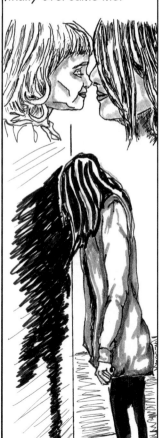

I stayed there for almost an hour trying to gather myself for the walk to my parking lot. I would have to pass people... patients...

...and God no, maybe even colleagues.

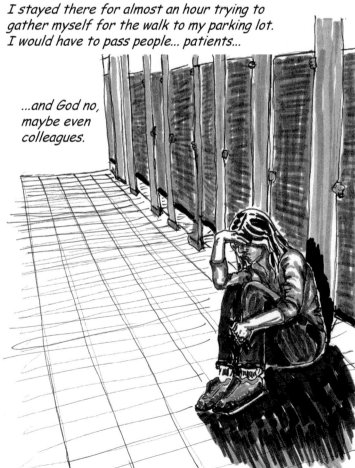

fig. 4.28

I lay awake again on Saturday night. I enjoyed some family time on Sunday. It was hard to look at my mom without hearing the girl's screams for her mother. There would be no answer.

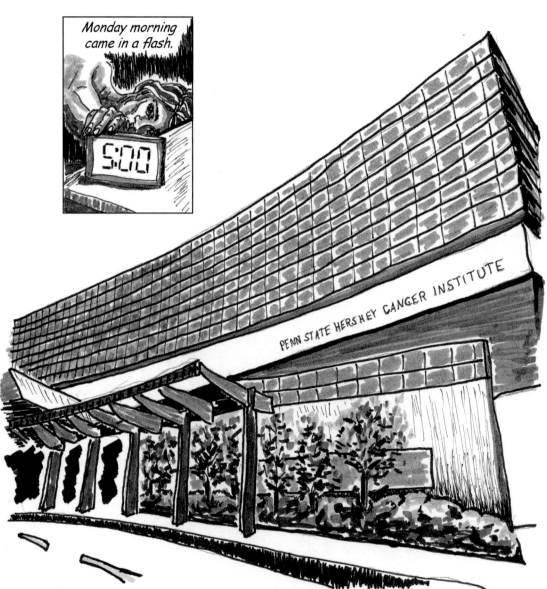

Monday morning came in a flash.

5:00

PENN STATE HERSHEY CANCER INSTITUTE

The sun was just starting to rise as I walked in to the hospital to begin a new week. I sighed and thought, "Vita perseverat." *Life goes on.*

Comics and the Iconography of Illness

- - - - -

IAN WILLIAMS

Introduction

In this chapter I aim to examine the depiction of disease, trauma, or suffering in comics, as well as to ask how the medium might create new knowledge and contribute to the bank of available images that inform our collective conceptions of illness and healthcare—what Sander Gilman calls the "iconography of illness."[1] I will focus specifically on the comics memoir of illness, what Green and Myers have termed the "graphic pathography," a direct descendant of the first autobiographical comics born of the West Coast counterculture of 1970s America.[2]

There seems to be a propensity among comics scholars to dissociate their fandom from their academic writing, so as to maintain the appearance of a detached analytical viewpoint. I have yet to meet a comics scholar, however, who is not enthusiastic about comics or else clearly in love with the medium. I will admit something up front: comics fascinate me. And in keeping with the personal tone of the writing in this volume, I will weave into the argument an account of how my interest in comics—and, latterly, my making comics—has allowed me to articulate my own experience of mental health problems (a subject that, as a health professional, I had previously been unwilling to discuss).

As a child I loved now-classic British children's comics, such as *The Beano* and *The Dandy*, but the first time I got really excited about comics was upon reading Issue 16 of *Dracula Lives*. A few years later I found the (also now-classic) UK comic *2000AD* profoundly exciting, freighted as it was with a 1970s dystopian view of the approaching millennium. I never developed a taste for superheroes, and as an older adolescent I started to read imported or reprinted editions of American underground comics, particularly the work of Gilbert Shelton.[3] I was a relatively clean-living youth growing up in the North of England, but Shelton's tales of San Francisco drug culture provided the vicarious thrill of transgression, both in the antics of characters such as the Fabulous Furry Freak Brothers and in our own regular forays to buy the comics from seedy "alternative" book shops that seemed to specialize in pornography and occult literature.

By the time I went to medical school at the age of 17—medicine is an undergraduate subject in the United Kingdom—my reading matter of choice was the outrageous adult comic *Viz*, a hilarious and puerile adult parody of the children's comics of my youth.[4] My years at university and my early adulthood were not without challenge: I had experienced recurrent bouts of mild to moderate depression since childhood, but during my mid-teens I developed an enervating obsessive-compulsive disorder (OCD), which I managed to keep hidden for many years out of fear that I would be ridiculed, medicated, or incarcerated. After working for some years as a junior doctor, I became a rural family physician in North Wales and undertook postgraduate studies in fine art, developing a side career as a painter and printmaker. My work was abstract and based on the landscape, which is important in Welsh culture for both poetic and political reasons.

Looking for a way to combine art and medicine, I enrolled in a master's degree program in medical humanities. I had expected to write my thesis on "medical" fine art, but before long I realized the link lay in the graphic novels I had begun to devour. Brian Fies's *Mom's Cancer* inspired me to write about medical narrative in comics and graphic novels. It soon became apparent that there were many authors who were putting their experience of healthcare and illness into comics form and that the comics memoir of illness—"graphic pathography"—constituted an important genre within comics. I found so many relevant works that I decided to create a website, which I called Graphic Medicine, and to post the notes made for my thesis there.[5]

Setting up the website changed my life and led me to discover my vocation. It soon became apparent that I was not alone in my interest in comics and medicine. One of the first people to contact me via the website was Michael Green, author of a previous chapter in this book. More introductions followed, and it became obvious that a number of people were interested in the interface between comics and medicine. Michael, Susan Squier, MK Czerwiec, and I met for the first time in London in 2010 at the first International Conference on Comics and Medicine, of which I was the lead organizer. Yearly conferences, published papers, and this book series have followed. The focus of Graphic Medicine so far has generally been on illness narratives in comics, but the rich visual dimension of the medium is surely as important as its diegesis.

The Visual Depiction of Illness

The consideration of visual depictions of disease in painting and photography is a worthwhile exercise with which to explore cultural ideas surrounding illness and healthcare, as Kimberly Myers reported in an earlier chapter. But as Kimberly points out, the analysis of fine art can be daunting: as a society we tend to lack adequate language with which to describe the visual, and we often resort to similes in our attempts to articulate what we perceive. Few of us command the intimidating argot of fine art criticism, and those of us from a healthcare background often find it rather alien to the pragmatic language of the clinic.

With comics, however, we seem to know a good visual narrative when we see one: as Chris Ware suggests, "you don't blame yourself for not 'getting' a comic strip—you usually blame the cartoonist."[6] This is not to say that we all read comics the same way or that meaning is immediately transparent. Comics may, however, invite engagement in cases where fine art might not. Graphic pathographies are rich in metaphor and visual depictions of illness and so are inherently engaged with the issues of healthcare. As Alan Radley states, "Whatever is shown about illness inevitably concerns medicine, whether this occurs by virtue of its presence or by virtue of its absence in the image."[7]

The imaging of diseased bodies remains central to medicine for both diagnostic and educational purposes, being an important way in which healthcare professionals learn and think about disease as well as document its effects on the body. Images help structure the schemata of illness within the mind of the clinician, who builds a mental catalogue of clinical signs and presentations against which the presenting appearances can be judged. Atlases of clinical signs serve as diagnostic aids, and modern imaging techniques offer the chance to visualize the interior of the body as well as the surface, further objectifying the body and enhancing the idea that the "truth" about the body can be obtained through technology and digital representation. These images require specialized knowledge for interpretation: "[t]he trained physician, taught to see fragments as signifying the whole, sees the essential link between the images, the disease and the patient."[8] Both this knowledge and the ability to make and interpret medical images of the body's interior give the physician tremendous power.

The mental frameworks of visual knowledge that healthcare professionals assemble during their training and work might admit more than pathology into their structure: no one is immune to media portrayals of their chosen vocation or immune to prevailing cultural attitudes toward such issues as gender roles, disability, or sexuality. We may not actually be aware of these influences, and this "not being aware" may be problematic for a couple of reasons. Firstly, we may be relying on knowledge we perceive to be "objective" but that is, in fact, highly subjective and influenced by our own cultural upbringing. Secondly, while these schemata might admit much subjective information from our own lives, they may not admit very much from the lives of our patients. If we are comparing patients to our own internal "ideal," we are likely to find them "abnormal," or at least a "variant" of normal. One way around these issues is to use popular media—such as comics—to approach the discussion of "the normal," stereotypes, or prejudice. Some effort should be made to incorporate into our thinking the wide range of "real life" appearances we actually encounter in day-to-day life as well as in the clinic.

Images do not just "mirror" the world; they help build it.[9] The proliferation of image-based media has also ensured that iconographic representations of health, illness, and disease have become increasingly important in Western societies.[10] These representations help construct the illness stereotypes that influence the way in which a condition is viewed by others[11] as well as the patient's experience of the condition. The self-picturing of suffering is a relatively new phenomenon that expanded in the twentieth century due to the availability of suitable media, such as photography. In constructing new visual styles of suffering and illness, therefore, the authors of graphic pathographies might be subtly altering the discourse of health and the social mediation of illness outside of the clinic.

The Iconography of Illness in Comics

The word "iconography" refers to the use of images and symbols to portray a subject, movement, or ideal. Most generally, the icon that Gilman refers to is the sign "that represents objects through a relationship of similarity by exemplifying some property associated with the object."[12] It is both simplification and generalization: its properties and features are important in defining what is signified. Comics images work as icons. Figures and faces are often a simplification of reality, yet we read them as a signification of "real" events happening to a "real" person. Meaning is enhanced and sensation intensified by exaggeration of posture and expression or by use of emanata (lines or words that protrude from a person or object "to show what's going on" or to "reveal internal conditions").[13]

The panel from *Monsters* by Ken Dahl (a pseudonym for Gabby Schulz) shows the author waking up with a lover, convinced that he has given her genital herpes (fig. 5.1).[14] Dahl portrays his feelings in the rictus of his face, the forehead beaded with sweat, the clenched hands, and the hole caved into his chest. The bug eyes with divergent pupils indicate a "thousand-yard stare" that, when combined with the other signs, reads as intense anxiety. The herpes virions that emanate from his body signal the focus of his anxiety, and, in the context of the preceding sequence, we know that his feelings are driven by a huge regret over what has just taken place.

The author's iconography will depend on influences from art, personal observation, and consumption of other medically themed media, articulated in

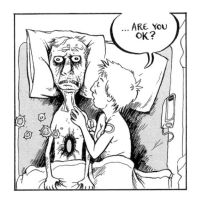

fig. 5.1
From Ken Dahl, *Monsters* (New York: Secret Acres, 2009).

a blend of intentional and unintentional signs. It will also depend on the skill and the style of the artist. As Roland Barthes notes, there is no drawing without style, without an apprenticeship.[15] Dahl is a talented artist who is able to convey meaning in a masterly way, where a less skilful comic artist might struggle to articulate what he is trying to say in graphic form and resort to an explanation of the narrative in text.

Ways of Showing

When drafting graphic pathographies, artists need to decide how to reinvent their sick bodies in ink or pixels and how visible to make their wounds. Before putting pen to paper, the making of a comic involves a decision-making process in how the artist should portray the illness. So important is the body in comics that Hilary Chute refers to the medium as a "procedure of . . . embodiment."[16] Similarly, Lisa El Refaie describes how "producing multiple drawn versions of the self entails an explicit engagement with physicality," and she uses the term "pictorial embodiment" (drawing upon the phenomenological work of Maurice Merleau-Ponty and Drew Leder) in order "to capture the different ways in which graphic memoirists' sense of self is linked with the act of visually representing their bodily identities."[17]

This drawing of one's own wounds has an ethical dimension: as Radley puts it, "to portray oneself visually, especially if one bears the visible marks of disease or its treatment, is to challenge assumptions about the scope or claims to health to which the sick are entitled."[18] He asks what role the portrayal of the "diseased-but-normal" self might play in the view of the healthy toward the sick, and he suggests that such images might help establish (however tentatively) a "viable way of living in the world."[19] Making autobiographical comics is a type of symbolic creativity that helps form identity—a way to reconstruct the world, placing fragments of testimony into a meaningful narrative and physically reconstructing the damaged body.

In order to examine these different ways of showing illness, then, I shall divide this section into three areas. The first group of problems one could call The Manifest, where the signs of illness or scars of treatment are visibly scripted on the body. The second group includes conditions that are only intermittently manifest or in which the psychological suffering outweighs the physical stigmata, that is, The Concealed: conditions that may not be noticed by, or are hidden from, the casual observer. The third category contains a group of conditions, such as mental illnesses, that are not inscribed on the skin of the patient—The Invisible—but are felt or produce psychological suffering. In such cases, the comics artist can use the iconographic flexibility of the form to make visible the effects of these conditions.

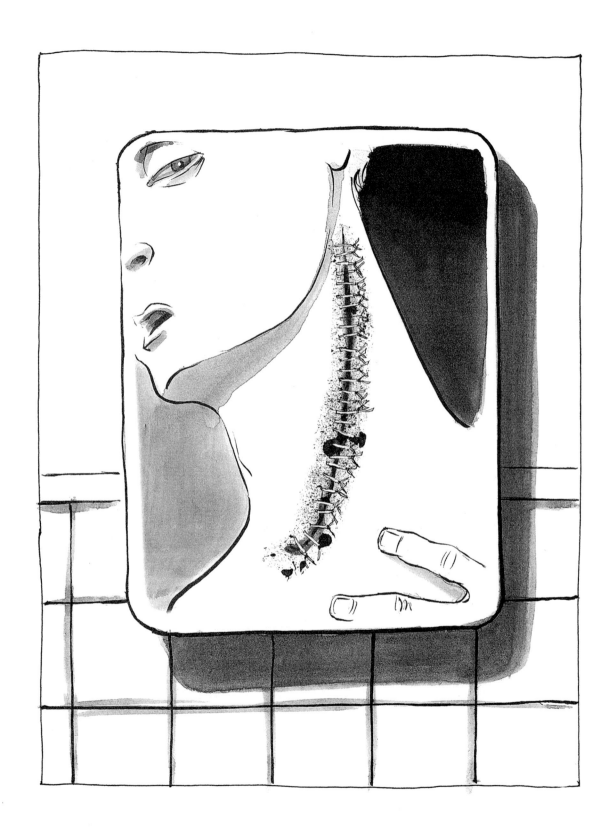

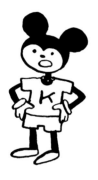

fig. 5.2 (OPPOSITE)
From David Small, *Stitches* (New York: W. W. Norton, 2009).

fig. 5.3
From Kaisa Leka, *I Am Not These Feet* (Helsinki: Absolute Truth Press, 2008).

This set of problems might appear to present the least trouble to autobiographical comics artists, who could simply choose to depict the stigmata of their illnesses as "realistically" as possible. Showing their wounds in graphic detail, however, anchors the experience as something alien to most readers and might risk the evocation of disgust or pity in the reader, reinforcing ideas that conflate sickness with ugliness and impotence. We dread being stigmatized: the most feared diseases are those that are "not simply fatal but transform the body into something alienating like leprosy and syphilis and cholera and . . . cancer."[20]

In *Stitches*, David Small's memoir about childhood cancer and family discord, he likens the wound that gives the book its title—the result of an operation for a thyroid tumor—to the laces of a "bloody boot" and draws the wound in realistic detail, set upon the neck of an iconically drawn self-portrait (fig. 5.2).[21] Small is emotionally and physically damaged by his parents, and this hurt comes through in the work. His unhappy mother did not love him, and his father, a radiologist, possibly induced the thyroid cancer by treating Small's asthma with X-rays.[22] In this panel, Small chooses to render his pain visually by placing the stitched wound at "center stage" and letting his partially reflected face fade into the background.

An alternative choice is to remove all detail and let the reader imagine the wound. The Finnish comics artist and politician Kaisa Leka subverts the usual portrayal of the sick body in her graphic novel *I Am Not These Feet*, which documents her decision to have her congenitally malformed feet amputated and replaced with high-tech prostheses. Portraying herself as a mouse, she employs the comics device of the anthropomorphic animal (fig. 5.3). Freed of the necessity for accurate self-representation and associations with the human form, anthropomorphic animals allow for the reconsideration of human stories in a different light.[23] The mouse avatar (literally) stands in for Leka, representing her altered body and reframing her experience. Scott McCloud, not uncontroversially, argues that the iconic simplification of cartoons encourages identification with the character: the simplification of facial features or bodily form means the drawing becomes a "vacuum into which our identity and awareness are pulled."[24] In other words, "[w]e don't just observe the cartoon, we become it."[25]

The simplified detail of Leka's lower legs and feet—two black lines with white loops at the base—frustrates our prurient curiosity and desire to see her deformity, allowing her to control the distance between author and reader. Deciding how much information to release, Leka withholds from us the emotional details, denying the graphic depictions the reader might desire (fig. 5.4). Rather than immersing us in a melodramatic autobiography, her restraint draws us in and fires our intrigue.

fig. 5.4
From Kaisa Leka, *I Am Not These Feet*
(Helsinki: Absolute Truth Press, 2008).

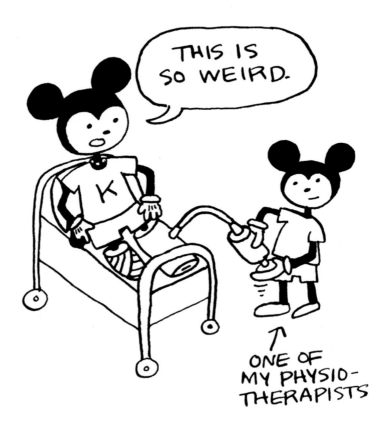

Leka's writing suggests that she feels better off without her feet, and, indeed, the book's title suggests that she rejects the idea of being defined by her impairment. Both the abstraction and the iconographic portrayal lessen the significance of Leka's deformity, in contrast to the excerpts in the next section by Dahl, who uses gross exaggeration to give an altogether different message.

The Concealed

I work in a sexual health clinic, dealing with infections and conditions whose hosts are usually keen to conceal. One of my favorite graphic novels, Dahl's *Monsters*— already discussed in Susan's chapter—uncovers a condition that causes immense psychological suffering to many people while rarely causing significant physical harm. In the following set of panels, Dahl uses a form of visual hyperbole to relay his feeling about contracting, living with, and spreading herpes. The book, an exercise in the grotesque that manages to yield important clinical and emotional information, is a semi-fictional memoir in which the author signals his own self-disgust by drawing himself as an oozing bag of infection—a vessel holding disease and, therefore, an extension of the disease (fig. 5.5).[26]

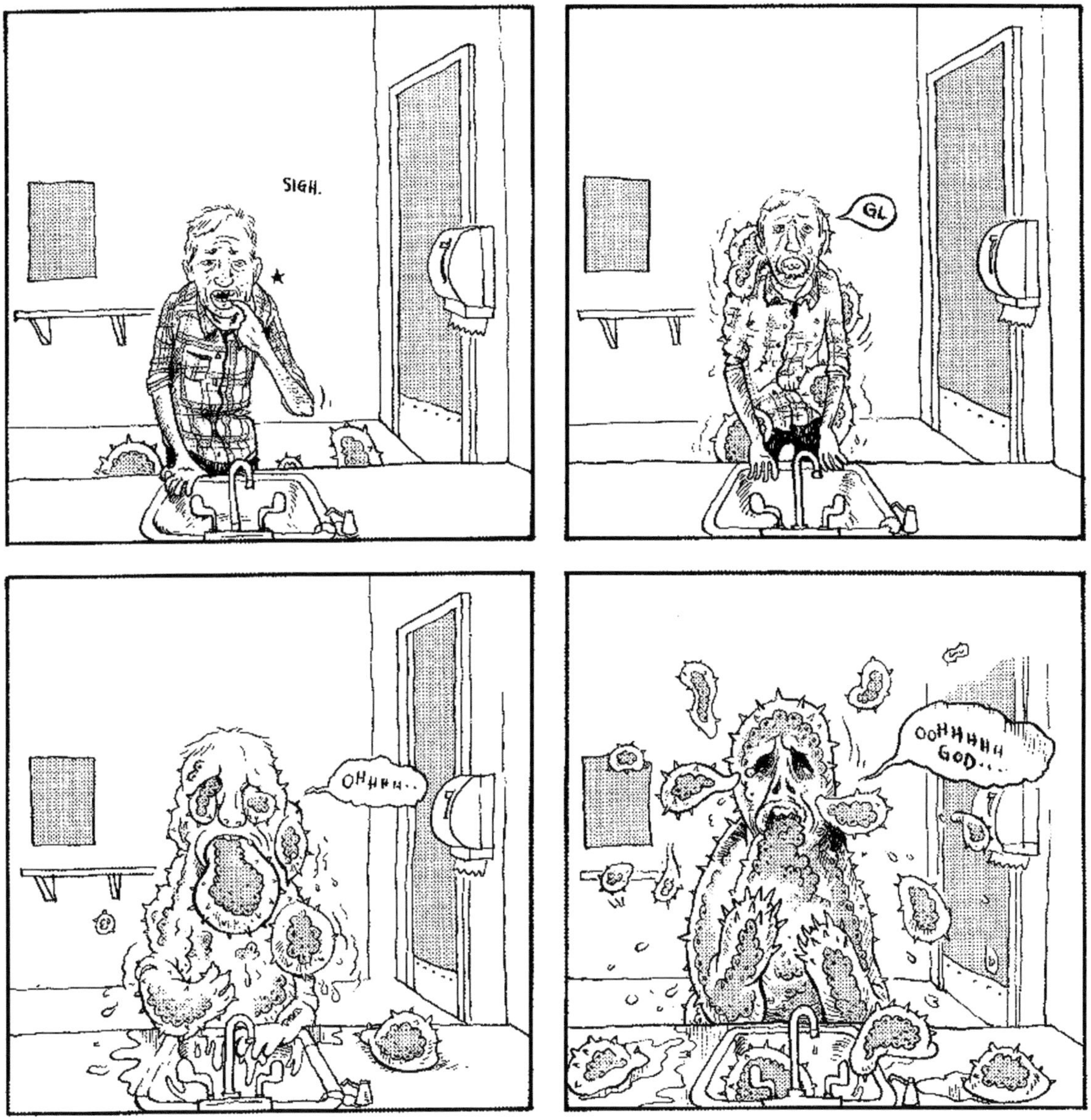
SIGH.
GL
OHHHH...
OOHHHHH GOD...

fig. 5.5
From Ken Dahl, *Monsters* (New York: Secret Acres, 2009).

At this point in the book, the protagonist, Ken, has been labeled as diseased and so has trawled the internet for images. "Have you ever done an internet search for 'herpes'?" he asks the reader. "It's like something out of a monster movie."[27] The codification of illness, according to Gilman, works on two levels: the first level is the "social construction of categories of disease"[28]—in this case herpes, which is represented on the internet by horrendous pictures of florid infection. Such terrible sights occasionally present themselves in clinics but cannot be said to constitute the "typical" presentation of the infection, which is rather less dramatic. In

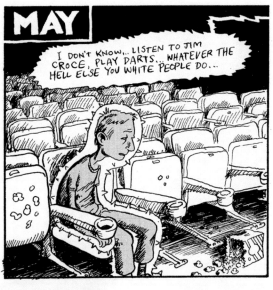

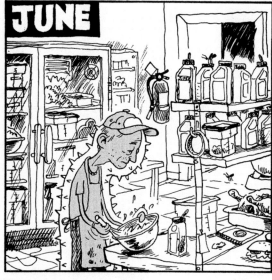

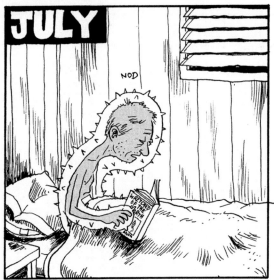

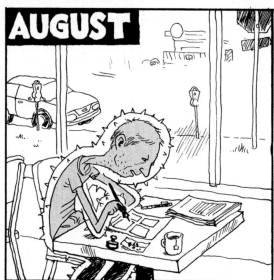

fig. 5.6
From Ken Dahl, *Monsters* (New York: Secret Acres, 2009).

fact, what I see in clinic represents the most dramatic end of the spectrum: the majority of infections go unnoticed, as "at least 80% of persons seropositive for HSV type-specific antibodies are unaware that they have been infected" and so do not seek medical advice.[29] The word "herpes," nevertheless, invokes in our minds the kind of horrific spectacle seen by Ken on his internet search, and it is the internalization of such images by groups labeled to be "at risk" that represents the second level of codification.[30] Dahl has internalized the iconography and drawn himself as a festering bag of virions, redefining his own self-perception. This series of panels, then, serves as both a commentary on and an example of the way in which images inform our ideas of disease.

With Ken as the herpes monster, Dahl iconically signals his pain and invokes our disgust and fear before leading the reader to a safer place by setting his terror in context, aided by some well-researched clinical information. Because *Monsters* is an amusing book, Dahl's excellently observed humor helps diffuse the fear invoked by the infection, as does his excellently articulated treatise on the stigma and social reverberations of what is, essentially, "just a skin rash."[31] As Susan asserts in her earlier chapter, *Monsters* sets the considerable social negotiations required to deal with this "skin rash" against wider biomedical and environmental problems.

Dahl uses physical space and the passing of time to signify his isolation and the potential contagion risk he thinks he poses by drawing himself surrounded by a viral envelope separating his "infected" body from "normal" society (fig. 5.6). He is using the diseased vessel simile again here, having been defined as a contaminated other.[32]

The concealed, then, can be revealed by the comics artist using various devices, including metaphor, exaggeration, simile, emanata, and the manipulation of physical space and time—all important comics techniques, some of which are unique to the medium.

The Invisible

There is a tradition within figurative art of showing various states of psychological distress, and over the centuries a lexicon of visual cues has been developed and remains powerful today. We know the classic pose of melancholia when we see it, because we recognize it from images we have internalized or observations of depressed people: slumped shoulders, the chin resting on the hand, the other in the lap, the expressionless face (see fig. 5.7). Is this pose some sort of "natural" posture to adopt when one is feeling melancholic, or is our behavior informed by the media we consume?

Writing about comics for my master's thesis motivated me to consider ways I might start to convey my own illness narrative and clinical experiences in comics form. The strips I started to make came out dark. I wanted to examine areas of medicine that seemed to be rarely discussed in clinical circles: abuses of power, frustration, and questionable behavior among healthcare staff. I started to put the strips online under a nom de plume, Thom Ferrier, and I slowly began to attract an audience. Looking back at early comic strips I drew, I am certain that I was not consciously thinking of Dürer when I drew my younger self during a long on-call shift, despairing at yet another summons by beeper (fig. 5.8).[33]

Conventions for visually displaying mental distress must have derived from numerous sources, including nineteenth-century psychiatric images, such as

fig. 5.7
Albrecht Dürer, *Melancholia I*, 1514. The
British Museum.

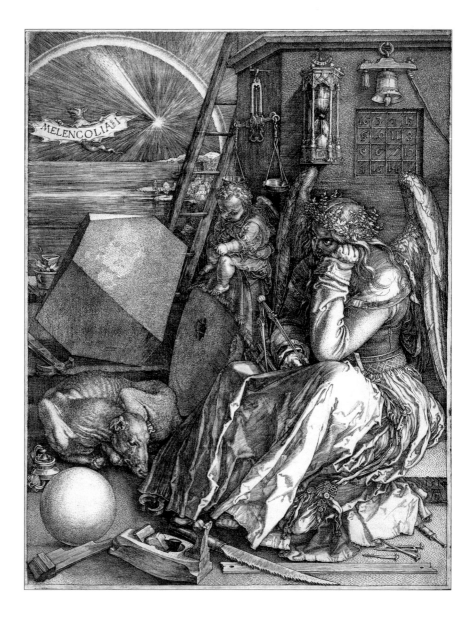

the photographs of mentally ill women in the *New Iconography of the Salpêtrière* (*Nouvelle iconographie de la Salpêtrière*), a journal that ran from 1888 to 1918, compiled initially by the neurologist Jean-Martin Charcot.[34] Along with other psychiatrists in his time, Charcot understood mental illnesses as "biological malfunctions that could be diagnosed on the basis of external physical indicators, especially facial expressions."[35] These conventions are still used in representations of the mentally ill in pharmaceutical advertising or photographic reportage, where they serve a diagnostic and naming function.[36]

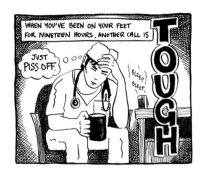

fig. 5.8
From Thom Ferrier, *Disrepute*
(Llanrhaeadr, Wales: Graphic Medicine, 2012).

The medium of comics uses and extends the language of classical art in signaling mood states using an expressionist mix of posture, expression, and visual metaphor, while also having the advantage of narrative text with which to fortify the effect. Examples of this can be seen in *Marbles: Mania, Depression, Michelangelo, and Me*, Ellen Forney's graphic account of her own bipolar illness. The book covers Forney's cycling mood level over a number of years. The visual conventions used to signal melancholy are seen in figure 5.9, in which her psychiatrist discusses medication changes.

When portraying deep depression, Forney draws herself lying on the sofa in the fetal position, wrapped in a blanket and hiding from the world (fig. 5.10). If it was not for the upholstered furniture, she could almost be a shrouded corpse, and while we know from the text that she is not, that simile must float in the corners of our consciousness.

These iconographic drawings work as metonyms for the underlying mood disorder, triggering a trace of the emotion in the reader. Comics demand reader participation—inviting readers to empathize with a subject by entering its world and seeing though its eyes—and enable the reader to gain insight from the vicarious experience. To portray mania, Forney uses emanata: spirals rising out of her spinning mind to signal confused thinking and arrows coming out of her mouth to signal pressure and volume of speech (fig. 5.11).

There is a lot going on in this image, and much of it would be cumbersome to put into words. One striking attribute is that the interlocked panels incorporate a flashback and an imagined scenario. Adrielle Mitchell, writing about graphic memoirs, notes that "planes of reality can coexist in the diegetic space of a comic—daily life, fantasy, spirit world, dream-space, myth, historical past, allegory, metaphor, metonym."[37] This facility, so full of potential for the portrayal of mental illness, is also used in a work that holds special significance for me: Justin Green's groundbreaking tale of neurosis and Catholic guilt, *Binky Brown Meets the Holy Virgin Mary*, an account of the author's experience of a religious form of OCD. In the panel reproduced here, we see the eponymous hero, Green's alter ego Binky Brown, imagining himself naked in a landscape populated with phallic trees (fig. 5.12).

Green spatially maps the "pecker rays" that Binky perceives to emanate from his penis and from other phallus-shaped body parts. Binky is compelled to keep the rays from pointing at religious statuary, in order to avoid blasphemy and sin. It seems unlikely that Binky actually sees the rays—OCD does not usually cause visual hallucinations—but he may picture them in his mind's eye or simply sense them to be invisibly present. Nevertheless, they seem real. This tortured divide between rational logic (the rays cannot really exist) and obsession (the rays are there, nonetheless) is a common feature of the condition. Similarly, Binky probably does not see his own feet and fingers as phalluses; rather, he associates their

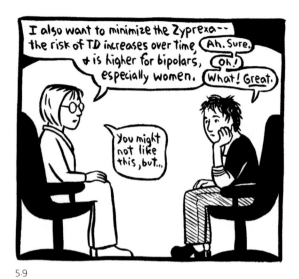

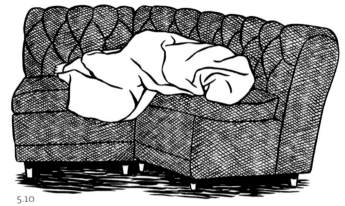

5.9

5.10

figs. 5.9–5.10
From Ellen Forney, *Marbles* (New York:
Gotham Books, 2012).

elongated shape as having the same phallic power as a penis, and so Green represents them metonymically.

Before I rediscovered comics I had never discussed my OCD publicly and, indeed, had hardly ever discussed it in private. Although my illness did not feature the transmission of "pecker rays," many of Binky's experiences did resonate with my own, and reading Green's comic encouraged me to try to express my own story in visual form. I had been experimenting with various methods of representing the effects that I experienced as a form of viral thought proliferation, with rapidly forming connections between unlinked propositions—"if I do this, that will happen"—which would then congeal into a rigid framework, limiting my actions and tying up my logic in an agonizing paralysis. Like Green's, my obsession was focused on religion. My infected adolescent logic was bound up in ideas of luck, spiritual contamination, and magic, so (years later and no longer bound by such tormented reasoning) I used the Sefiroth of the Kabbala to provide the framework for a drawing that attempts to convey my experience, with the intention of using it in my graphic novel, *The Bad Doctor*, a fictional story that draws on certain aspects of my own experience. This image would, of course, require some explanation if presented without the context of an ongoing narrative about OCD—as, indeed, would the example from *Binky Brown*. In the end, I used a slightly different version of the drawing as part of a series of tableaux that punctuate the book (fig. 5.13).

Our motives, I suspect, are often opaque to ourselves, and attempting to write about such complex matters further complicates the enterprise, but there seems to me to be an aspect of performance in what I have done. I suspect that in rendering my experience into a series of images, I am striving for a sense of ownership over

fig. 5.11
From Ellen Forney, *Marbles* (New York: Gotham Books, 2012).

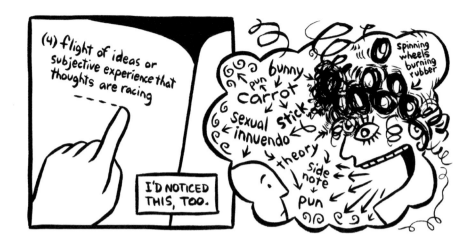

my condition—to transform it from a stigmatizing mental defect and source of shame to me as a medical professional into something of mystery and beauty.

Official Versus Unofficial Iconography

I find comics' potential to show lived perceptual experience exciting, charged with possibilities for the deepening of dialogues about health and illness. Medicine is a discourse with a highly developed and specialized technical language. Textbooks, guidelines, and verbal discussion among healthcare professionals could be seen as constituting the "official" language of healthcare: sanctioned by authority, peer reviewed, and packed with "objective" and "evidence-based" propositions. It is through these avenues of approved knowledge that the discourse exerts its power. The visual aspects of the discourse are mediated though an analogous official iconography that shows how sick people should look and helps distinguish the "normal" from the "abnormal." The marks of disease on the body are appropriated by medical photographers or illustrators; positioned in "neutral," anatomically "correct" positions and in the "correct" light; and captured in photographs or drawings. Any sense of the individual is removed by cropping off the head, isolating the body part, or blacking out the eyes.

Graphic memoirs of illness, on the other hand, stem precisely from the need to express oneself and, possibly, to challenge the "medical" authority from which the author feels excluded. This "unofficial" iconography of medicine emerges from any graphic work that creates new ways of representing disease, whether or not the author necessarily means to challenge the official knowledge: subjective interpretations, even when explaining conventional wisdom, may provide new insights. The independent comics artist may create an original iconography that transmits the raw veracity of lived experience.

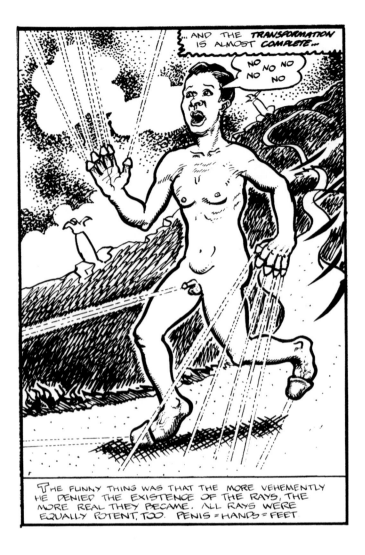

The cutting edge of graphic medicine could be said to exist in the hand-lettered, hand-produced 'zines found at small-press fairs and in self-produced web comics. Authors such as Andrew Godfrey, who has cystic fibrosis (CF), are using comics to portray their truths about living with terminal illnesses. Godfrey's untutored drawing style and scrawled handwriting add a certain lo-fi authenticity to his *CF Diaries*, while the author's status as a sick person allows him to explore areas such as isolation, narcissism, and facing death (fig. 5.14). Godfrey often portrays himself as looking sicker than he in fact is, railing against the poster-boy romanticism used in awareness-raising campaigns, which seem awash with mixed visual messages. The condition is serious and needs financial support, yet thickened secretions, fatty stools, and infertility are unsexy details that risk repulsing

fig. 5.13
Comic by author.

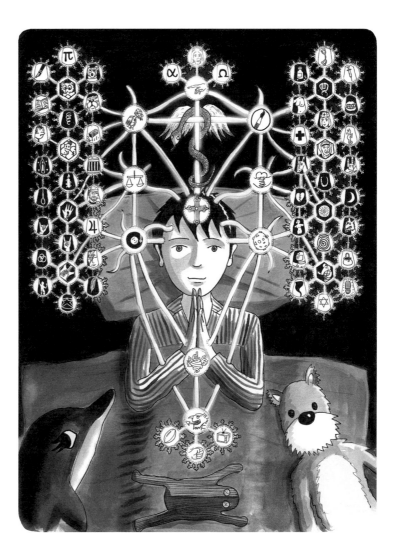

those uninvolved "healthy" people who are confronted with a host of needy causes vying for their donations. A web trawl for images of CF is as likely to show glamorous celebrities who support "CF awareness" as it is to show people who have CF themselves. Most health-informational images represent the body in classical medical illustrative form, showing thickened secretions in the airways and generally focusing on the lungs, even though the condition affects the whole body. The effects of the condition upon the organs of reproduction—infertility, surely a significant factor for those affected—are rarely mentioned.

 The fact that the author is living with a terminal illness gives *The CF Diaries* authority. Godfrey rejects sympathy and, in doing so, reestablishes his identity as someone living an altered—yet equally meaningful—life course. One of

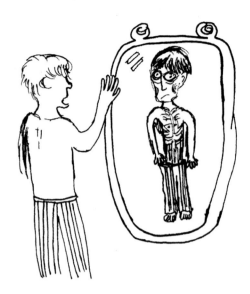

fig. 5.14
From Andrew Godfrey, *The CF Diaries*
(Bristol: Sicker Than Thou Industries,
2011).

Godfrey's influences, the performance artist, comic, and poet Bob Flanagan, notoriously rejected received ideas about how the "sick" should behave by incorporating feats of extreme masochism into his performances, such as acts that included hammering a nail though his penis. Flanagan used self-inflicted pain to challenge notions of the passively suffering sick body.[38] The practice of BDSM (bondage, discipline, and sadomasochism) worked for Flanagan to regain some control over his body—for what do we fear in illness, if not loss of bodily control? Graphic memoirs of illness might derive from a similar need to regain control over one's body, to reclaim it from the hands of the healthcare professionals. If we cannot quarantine disease, as Gilman has it, by imaging it or showing the other as its bearer, we might at least ameliorate our anxiety by owning our own conditions.

What is captivating about the best graphic pathographies is that they contain precisely the information that is left out of or never considered for inclusion in textbooks. Some, to be sure, are well researched and include detailed anatomical and pathological illustrations that would be at home in a textbook, but they often go further—depicting emotion and feeling, tackling the taboo or the liminal. The amount of information and meaning in a comic depends on new representations of illness that have not been previously seen in textbooks or "lay documents," such as informational leaflets for patients. Comics excel at articulating subjective notions or layered, equivocal meanings. If there is a hierarchy of style with regard

graphic medicine
manifesto

132

to the visual portrayal of the sick, then new truths are often to be found in the most raw and visually unpolished of self-publications.

Conclusions

A comic's power is related to image and text, choice of structure, story and backstory, and the cultural positioning of the medium itself. Authors of graphic memoirs of illness, by depicting their conditions and experiences, create valuable new knowledge, which informs the iconography of illness. Their work deserves wider recognition within the healthcare professions and within academia. While comics are knowledge and theory, graphic medicine should also open a debate with visual studies in order to examine healthcare comics from numerous angles.

Medicine is constructed around a taxonomy of diseases in which differentiation and categorization of conditions are conducted partly in visual terms, yet practitioners are often blind to the assumptions made in their mental schemata or textbook depictions of "typical" disease presentations. Visual assessments of the sick are linked to deep-seated, culturally accrued attitudes within the observer that may also be unacknowledged or unconscious. These latent attitudes may be addressed by the consideration and discussion of images, along with the meanings inherent within them, or by the reading and appraisal of comics and graphic novels. Indeed, healthcare professionals *are* reading comics, and while this influence may work initially at a "grassroots level," schools of healthcare and peer-reviewed journals are beginning to investigate and use the medium. One of the implicit aims of this volume is to encourage and widen the acceptance of the medium within clinical practice.

Comics artists who portray themselves autobiographically face many decisions in how to portray themselves in sickness, although they may not be aware of the decisions they are making or the effects that those decisions have in subtly reshaping the cultural model of disease and disability. Artists use a variety of innovative and traditional visual codes to express their illness experiences, which may vary depending on whether the problem is manifest, concealed, or invisible. Their powerful depictions might be said to belong to the radical, unofficial iconography of healthcare, of which the medium of comics is, as yet, an underused source.

· · · · · · · · ·

FIGURES ON
FOLLOWING PAGES
▬ ▬ ▬ ▬ ▬ ▬

figs. 5.15–23
From Glyn Dillon, *The Nao of Brown*
(London: SelfMadeHero, 2012).
Courtesy of Glyn Dillon.

The following pages reproduce an extract from Glyn Dillon's masterpiece *The Nao of Brown*. Nao, a half-Japanese girl, who suffers from OCD, is plagued by intrusive thoughts of violence toward others, which she finds very distressing. Dillon articulates Nao's condition by means of an internal dialogue and the seamless blending of reality and fantasy in the images.

fig. 5.15

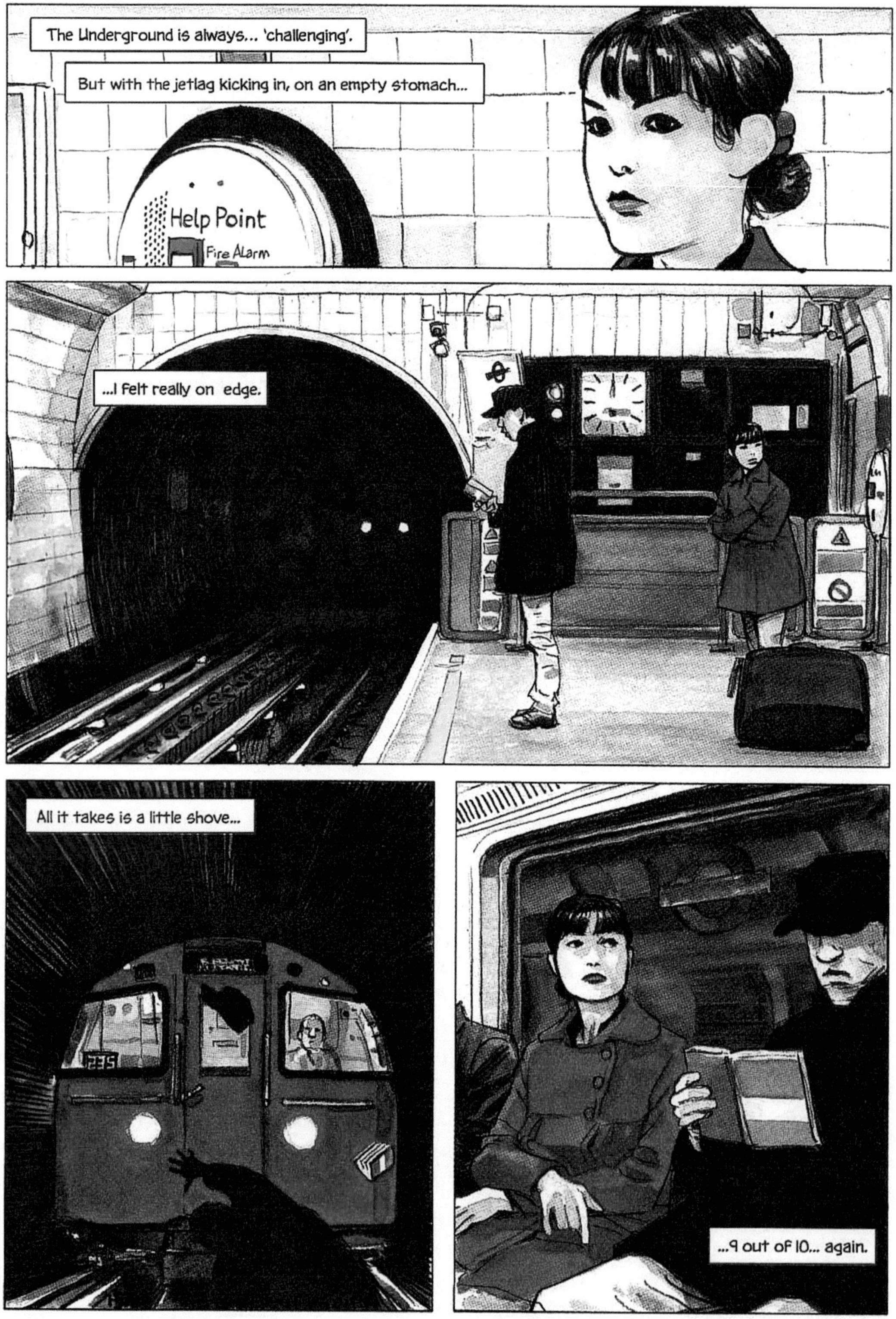
The Underground is always... 'challenging'.
But with the jetlag kicking in, on an empty stomach...
Help Point
Fire Alarm
...I felt really on edge.
All it takes is a little shove...
...9 out of 10... again.

fig. 5.16

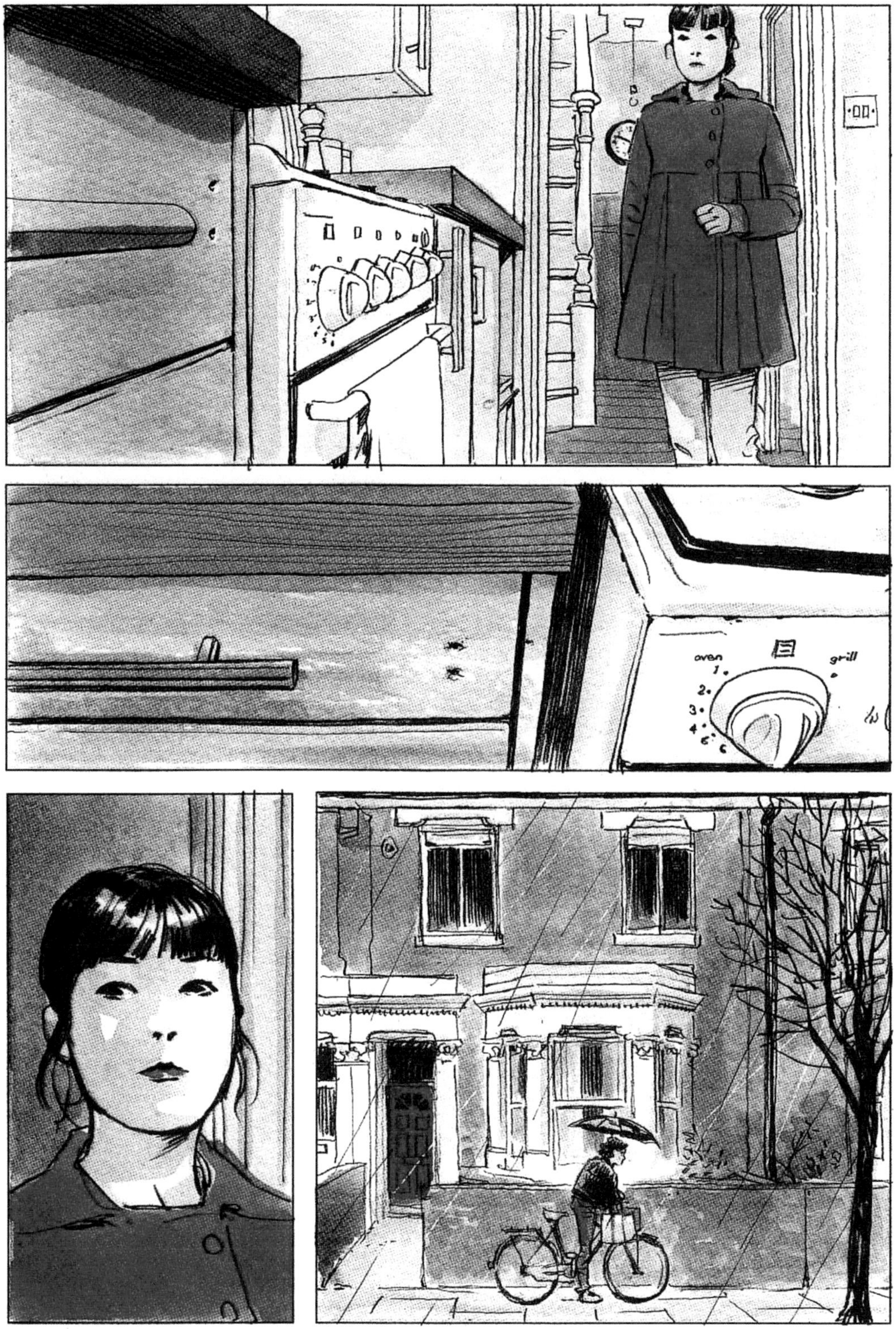
oven
grill

fig. 5.17

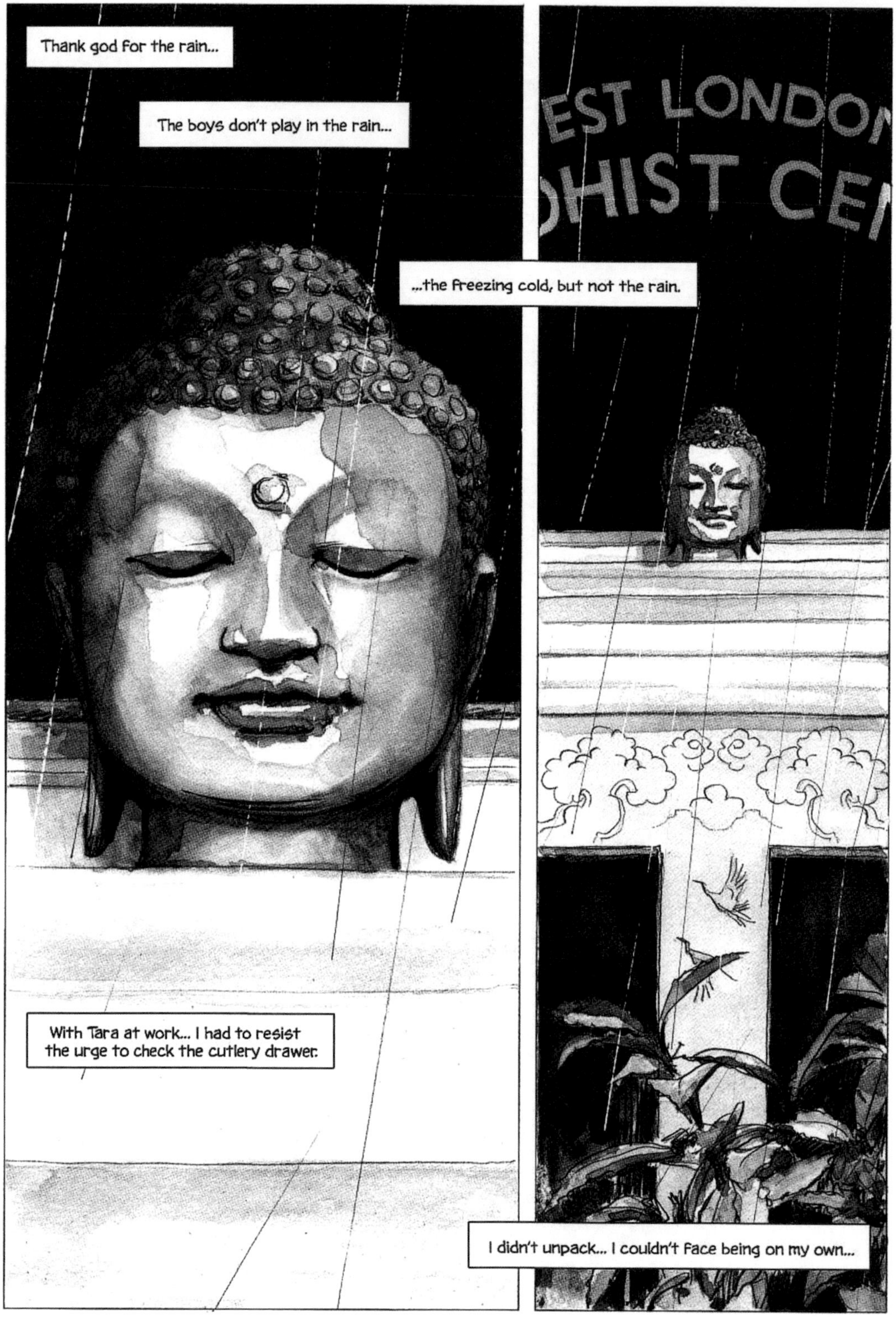
Thank god for the rain...
The boys don't play in the rain...
...the freezing cold, but not the rain.
EST LONDON
DHIST CEN
With Tara at work... I had to resist the urge to check the cutlery drawer.
I didn't unpack... I couldn't face being on my own...

fig. 5.18

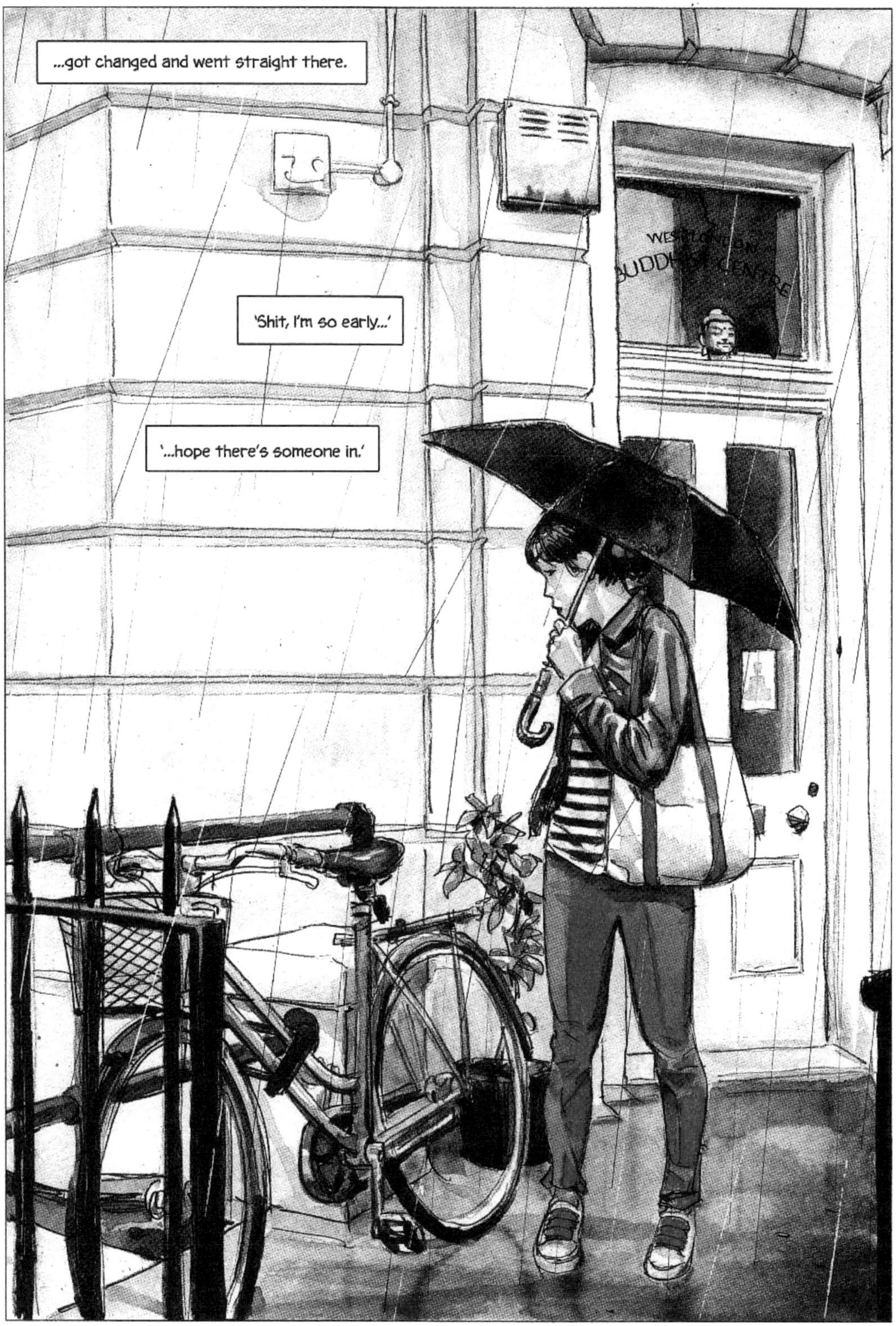
...got changed and went straight there.
'Shit, I'm so early...'
'...hope there's someone in.'

fig. 5.19

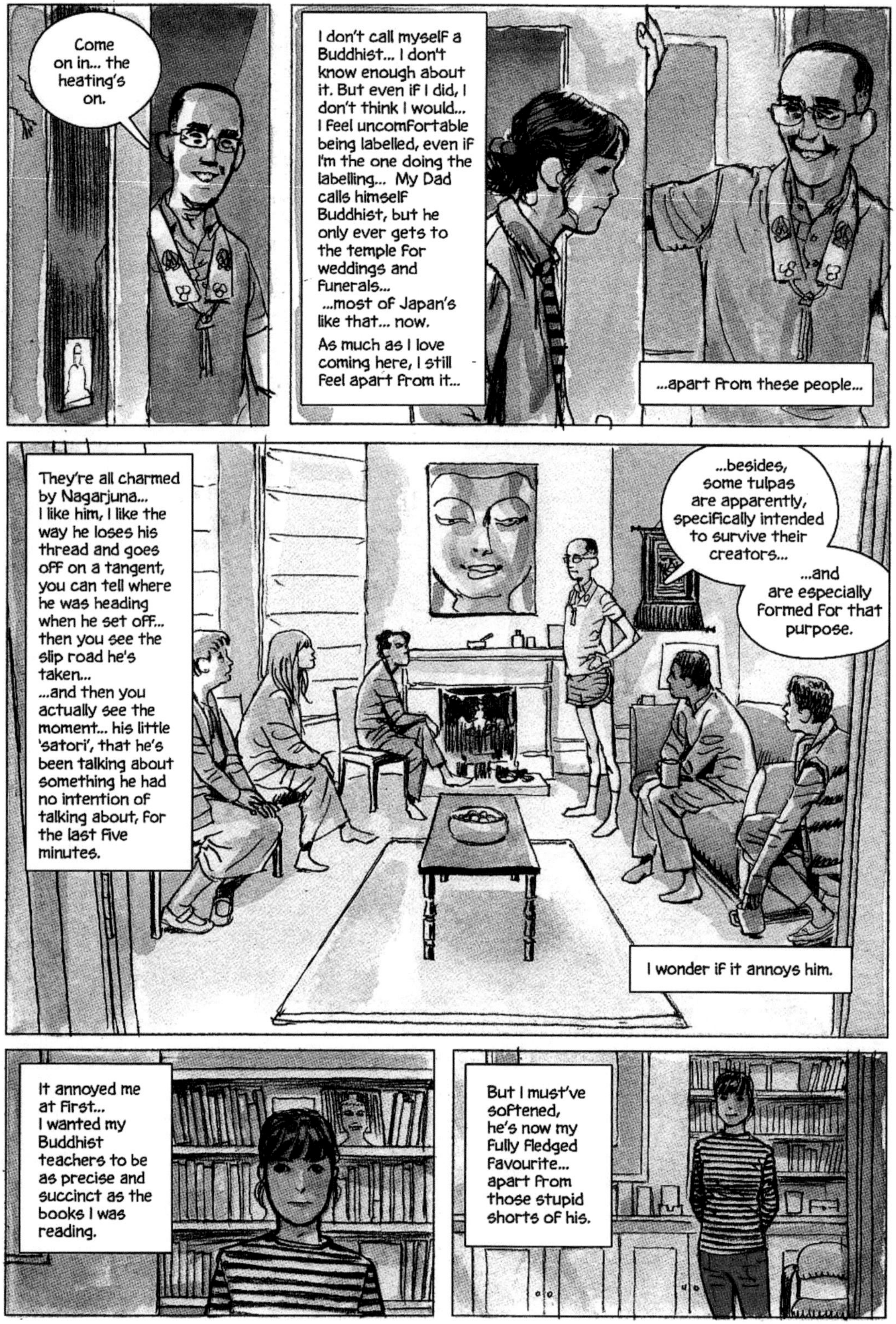

Come on in... the heating's on.
I don't call myself a Buddhist... I don't know enough about it. But even if I did, I don't think I would... I feel uncomfortable being labelled, even if I'm the one doing the labelling... My Dad calls himself Buddhist, but he only ever gets to the temple for weddings and funerals... ...most of Japan's like that... now.
As much as I love coming here, I still feel apart from it...
...apart from these people...
They're all charmed by Nagarjuna... I like him, I like the way he loses his thread and goes off on a tangent, you can tell where he was heading when he set off... then you see the slip road he's taken... ...and then you actually see the moment... his little 'satori', that he's been talking about something he had no intention of talking about, for the last five minutes.
...besides, some tulpas are apparently, specifically intended to survive their creators...
...and are especially formed for that purpose.
I wonder if it annoys him.
It annoyed me at first... I wanted my Buddhist teachers to be as precise and succinct as the books I was reading.
But I must've softened, he's now my fully fledged favourite... apart from those stupid shorts of his.

fig. 5.20

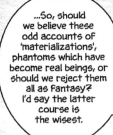
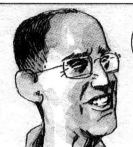
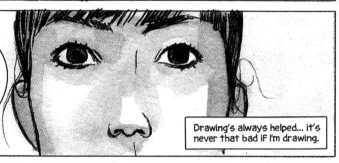

...So, should we believe these odd accounts of 'materializations', phantoms which have become real beings, or should we reject them all as fantasy? I'd say the latter course is the wisest.

And perhaps *getting on* is wiser still. How did we get on to that? Was that your fault, Linda?

So, we're going to split into two...

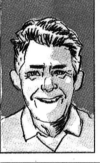
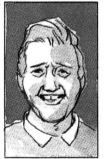
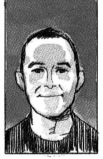
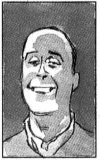

...those of you who want to have a go at Haiku stay in here with me and those of you who want to have a dabble with the brushes go with Ray. Then at eight we'll go downstairs for forty-five minutes' meditation.

Drawing's always helped... it's never that bad if I'm drawing.

Most of the men join me in heading for the end of the room with brushes and ink, only a few stay behind with the ladies to come up with something snappy in seventeen syllables.

The men who come here all seem really... well, nice, obviously Romantics... and one or two obviously gay.

...Dignaga, however, is a different story, he's got something about him, looks like an old punk or an ex-junkie, maybe it's his Shane MacGowan smile... and that 'doesn't suffer fools gladly' air he has about him...

The way he looks at me, I just feel stupid... I'm sure he knows I'm stupid... so naturally I dislike him... yet at the same time I feel the desperate need to please *him* more than anyone else.

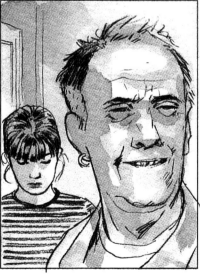
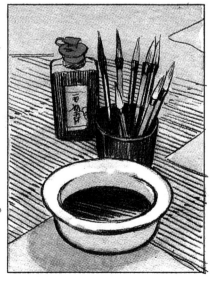

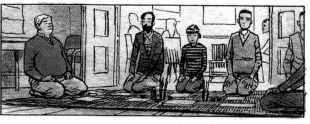

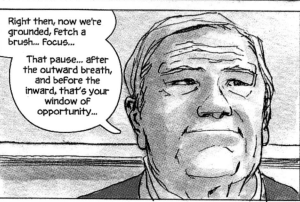

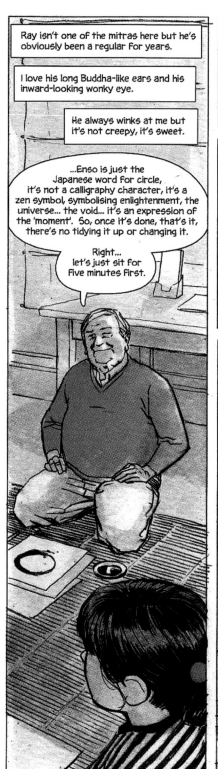

Ray isn't one of the mitras here but he's obviously been a regular for years.

I love his long Buddha-like ears and his inward-looking wonky eye.

He always winks at me but it's not creepy, it's sweet.

...Enso is just the Japanese word for circle, it's not a calligraphy character, it's a zen symbol, symbolising enlightenment, the universe... the void... it's an expression of the 'moment'. So, once it's done, that's it, there's no tidying it up or changing it.

Right... let's just sit for five minutes first.

Right then, now we're grounded, fetch a brush... Focus...

That pause... after the outward breath, and before the inward, that's your window of opportunity...

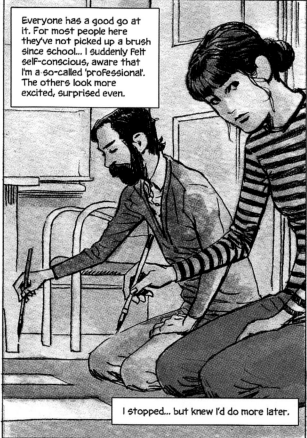

Everyone has a good go at it. For most people here they've not picked up a brush since school... I suddenly felt self-conscious, aware that I'm a so-called 'professional'. The others look more excited, surprised even.

I stopped... but knew I'd do more later.

fig. 5.21

fig. 5.22

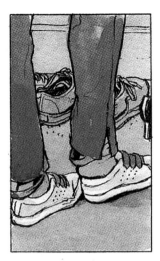

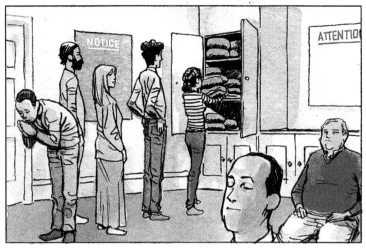

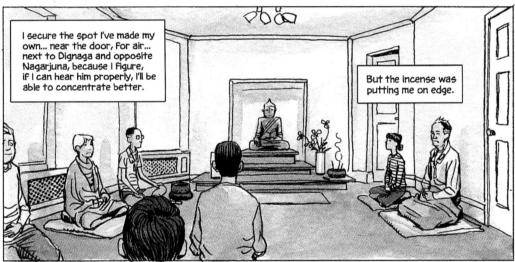

I secure the spot I've made my own... near the door, For air... next to Dignaga and opposite Nagarjuna, because I figure, if I can hear him properly, I'll be able to concentrate better.

But the incense was putting me on edge.

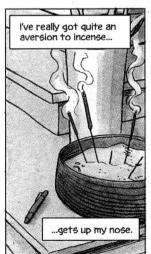

I've really got quite an aversion to incense...

...gets up my nose.

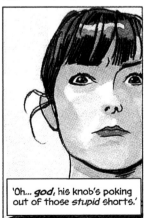

'Oh... *god*, his knob's poking out of those *stupid* shorts.'

'...again.'

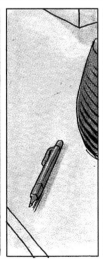

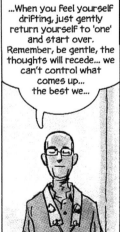

...When you feel yourself drifting, just gently return yourself to 'one' and start over. Remember, be gentle, the thoughts will recede... we can't control what comes up... the best we...

fig. 5.23

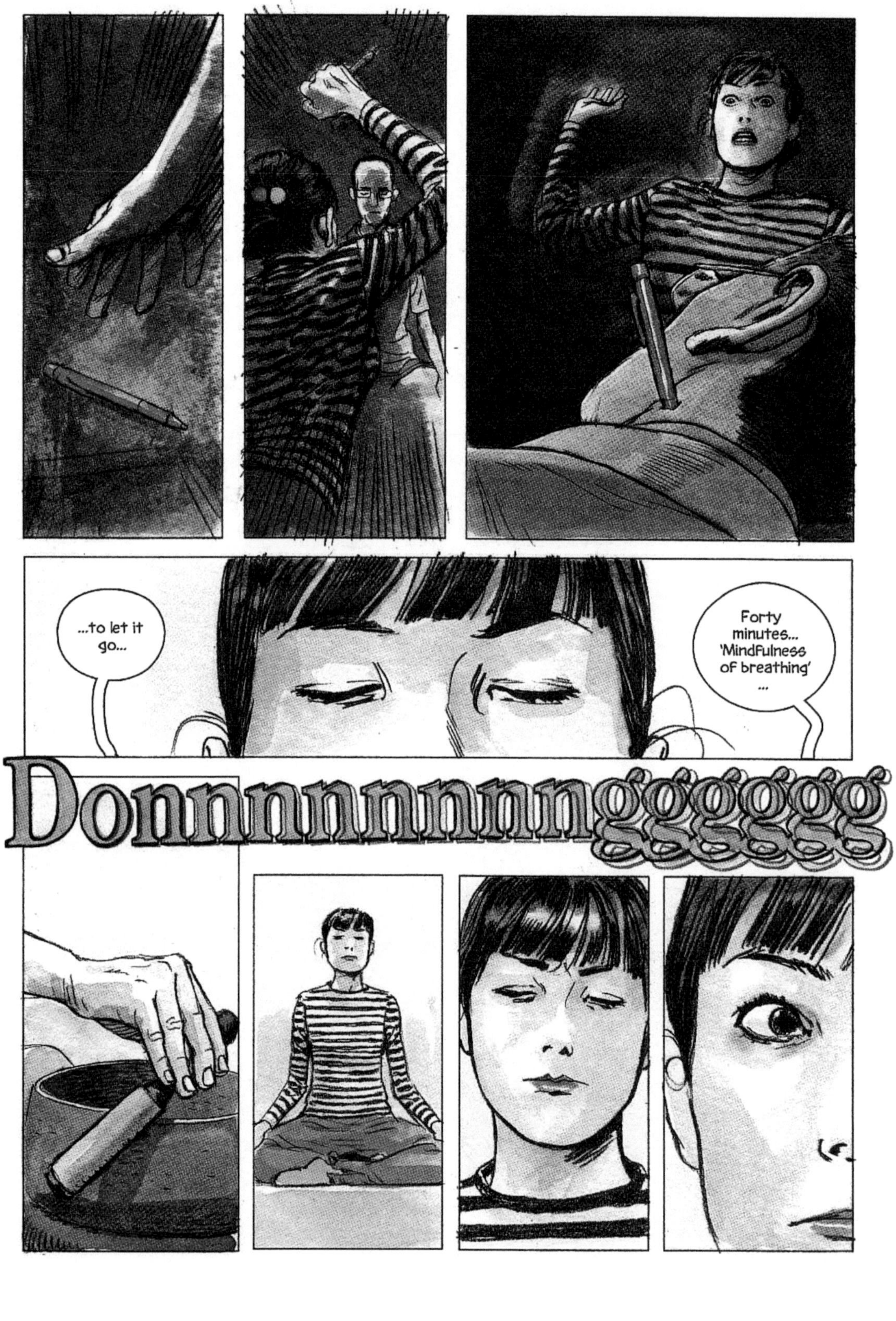
...to let it go...
Forty minutes... 'Mindfulness of breathing' ...
Donnnnnnnnnngggggg

The
Crayon
Revolution

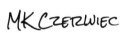

MK Czerwiec

There is a kind of impossible intimacy [in comics] especially when something is written and drawn by one person . . . as soon as you see someone's drawing and handwriting, you're given an insight into them.

—ART SPIEGELMAN, "AN EVENING WITH ART SPIEGELMAN AT THE CENTRAL LIBRARY," 2011

My Origin Story

I remember the exact moment I made my first comic. It was the spring of 2000. I was thirty-three years old. The comic happened mostly by accident the morning after a very difficult evening shift on the AIDS unit in Chicago where I worked as a nurse. Despite new and very promising antiviral medications, a beloved patient had just died. It had also recently become clear that, because of these new drugs, few patients with HIV needed to be hospitalized, so the AIDS unit where I worked would soon be closing.

This latter news was cause for celebration; the hospital, and the community it served, no longer needed a dedicated inpatient AIDS unit! I wanted to feel elated—some of my friends would perhaps survive the devastating plague—but I was ashamed to admit I was actually very sad. Losing the security and community of this AIDS unit felt like another death. I felt sad and anxious and ashamed that morning as I sat before a blank white piece of paper, trying to help myself look at this tangle of feelings.

During the time I worked as an AIDS nurse, before there were effective medications to cope with this disease, when nearly every new patient we would meet would likely die within a few months or years, I had first coped with stress by writing. But after a while, words were inadequate. Despite having no artistic training, and coming from a place of need, I started to paint. I used acrylic paint on panels of wood to make large and small folding screens as memorials to patients and friends who had died. (It occurs to me now that those panels were in some way precursors to my comics.)

But this day, the morning after this beloved patient had died and I was facing the loss of our AIDS unit, words alone and isolated images on screens or paper failed me. I sat staring at a piece of blank white paper at my old wooden drawing table. Not knowing what else to do, I drew a picture of myself in the top left corner of the paper. It was me, as I saw myself in that moment, nowhere near my best: dirty hair, glasses, old baseball hat, stained t-shirt, sad. Not knowing what to do next, and feeling as though at any second I might crumple the paper into a ball, throw it at the garbage can, and just give up, I wrote a few words above the drawing of myself. I wrote, "I feel miserable." Then I drew a box around the words and self-portrait. I had not started this exercise with the intention of making a comic; it had never occurred to me. Because there was one box in the upper left corner of an otherwise blank piece of paper, I drew another box next to the first. Staring at what I'd done, I thought about Lynda Barry's work. I remembered the weekly four-panel *Ernie Pook's Comeek* that I loved to read during my college years, and how Barry used comics to deal with painful subjects. What I didn't realize in that moment was that the empty space between two boxes in a comic, the gutter, takes a static state—in this case my sadness—and makes it do something, makes it go somewhere, anywhere, turning a static state into a story. The gutter space asks the question that was the favorite of the late oral historian Studs Terkel: "And then what happened?"[1]

In the next box, I started with the text. I wrote a few words about the causes of my pain. I drew a picture to accompany that text. I drew another box. I kept going. Nine boxes later, I found myself in a place of insight and, much to my surprise, hope. I liked what I'd done. Rather than crumpling it and tossing it into the trash, I wanted to put this piece of paper up on the wall as a testament to the important thing that had just happened.

The next day, I went to my drawing table and followed the same process, but this time with the intention of making a comic. And it worked again. So I kept it up.

Not until I was finishing graduate school in medical humanities and bioethics did I start contemplating what it was about creating comics that made them "work" for me as a nurse attempting to cope with challenging work experiences. What was it about drawing a succession of boxes filled with a few words and images that took me from that static state of despair to a new place of insight and hope? What was happening as I made a comic—and was it something unique to me or could others have this experience as well?

After graduation, armed with a few ideas about what I had started to think of as reflective drawing and the benefits it could hold for medical students, I developed a pilot seminar for Northwestern medical students—with the collaboration and guidance of Catherine Belling—called Drawing Medicine. Most of the content of this chapter has evolved from twice-yearly teaching that five-week seminar for the past five years. Teaching this seminar has convinced me of the truth that animates this essay: drawing a comic—which requires things we each already possess: words, a visual language, a writing implement, and a blank piece of paper—has enormous potential when used in the medical context.

Part 1: Why Don't We All Draw?

Once I realized how powerful drawing had been for me, and started thinking that it might also be helpful for others in healthcare, I wondered why many of us stop using drawing as a way of thinking, of processing our lived experiences. My quest for an answer took me back to early grade school.

For the past ten years, I have volunteered with a literacy group in Chicago called Sit Stay Read. The group's Guest Reader program provides me with the opportunity to regularly speak with grade-school students about drawing. When I ask first-grade students, "Who here is an artist?," figure 6.1 is what I generally see. Students are joyful, and they proudly celebrate their drawing by enthusiastically throwing their arms in the air. The teacher is happy too.

But when I go down the hallway to a fifth-grade classroom and ask the same question, "Who here is an artist?," I see something more like figure 6.2. There is hesitation and debate around the responses. One or two students will raise their hands. One student might be corrected by another next to him, and he will put his hand down. Other students might wish they could say they were artists, but they feel unworthy to say so. A few students might point to one student who "can draw." The teacher will often also point to that student as the "class artist."

What happens between first and fifth grades that causes children to stop drawing? There is an acknowledged phenomenon known as the "fourth grade slump." The term was coined to refer to a dip in literacy that happens around this age. E. Paul Torrance, in a 1967 report to the U.S. Department of Health, Education, and Welfare, expanded the use of the term to include a dip in children's creative development.[2] He states that by the time kids are in the fourth grade, "there is a rather severe decrement in almost all of the creative thinking abilities."

When I was young, I was not one of the kids who "could draw." I was one of the kids encouraged to *stop* drawing. We got the message that crayons were

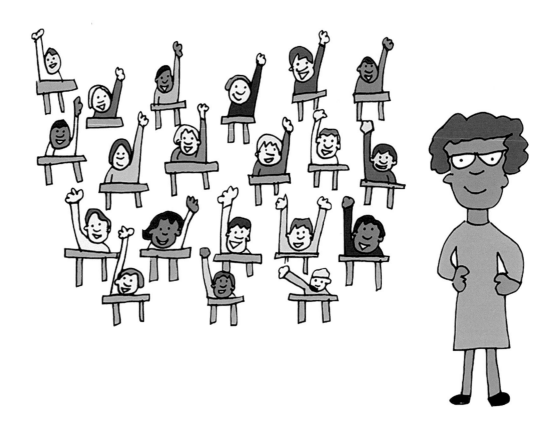

fig. 6.1
MK Czerwiec, *Happy Class*, 2012.

to be put away. No more coloring and drawing—we were to stick to words instead. Drawing as the expression of our ideas, thoughts, and learning was a childish thing to be left behind. Those who "could draw" were allowed to continue, but only as long as they still seemed to have what parents and teachers called "talent." Talent seemed to be defined in this context as the ability to realistically render objects beyond the expected ability for their age. As cartoonist Lynda Barry writes, "The rest of us were left wishing."[3]

And so we wrote our words. Yet those of us who were good with words were not the only ones who were allowed to continue using words. All students were required to improve their use of words to articulate their thoughts and ideas. Why did this attitude not apply to the use of images? What did we leave behind in fourth grade when most of us stopped drawing?

Barry has said, "If [I] had a 40-year-old person next to me and I had paper and markers and I said, let's make a picture, and that person was too scared to do it, we'd understand. If I had a four-year-old sitting next to me and she was too scared to do it, we'd be worried about her emotionally, right?"[4] Why is that? Why do we worry when a child is too afraid to draw but think it is perfectly acceptable, if not *the norm*, when an adult is?

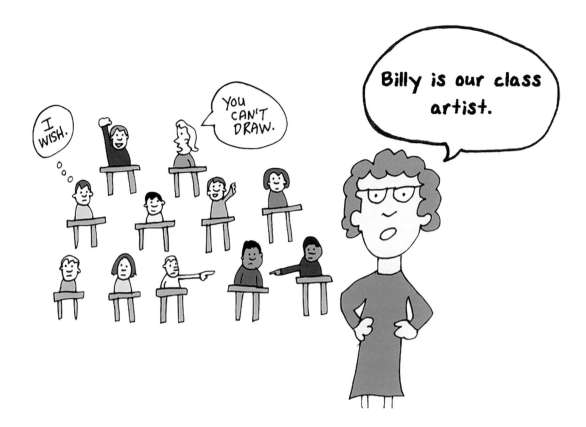

fig. 6.2
MK Czerwiec, *You Can't Draw*, 2012.

Part 2: The Power of the Crayon

After presenting to various groups on drawing comics—from those reticent fifth graders, to high-school students, to adults—one thing I have found is that crayons are the great equalizer. Despite the ubiquitous statements about "not being able to draw," every individual in every one of those groups knows what to do with a crayon, and they pick crayons up with gusto—particularly medical students. I tend to open every workshop or group activity by asking the participants to draw a self-portrait in crayon as a way to introduce themselves to the group. And what is revealed in this exercise is that every person already has a visual language of his or her own, whether it has been developed for years or whether it stopped in fourth grade. Author and illustrator Sarah Leavitt, creator of *Tangles: A Story About Alzheimer's, My Mother, and Me*, understands this. She said in a 2010 talk at Edmonton's Nonfiction Festival, "When people say they can't draw what they usually mean is, 'I cannot sit down in front of something and reproduce it realistically.' . . . I would actually say that 'good drawing' is being able to create a drawing that expresses an emotion, one that people can read, understand what you are trying to say, and are moved by it."[5] The easiest way for us to access this innate visual language seems to be with a crayon.

Bringing crayons back to the classroom is a great place to start. Once we have gone around the room in the drawing workshop, not one participant can now say he or she "can't draw" because we have seen that everyone can. Returning to drawing as an adult is about being willing to pick up wherever you left off and about embracing the visual language you already possess—rather than judging "talent." In a 2011 blog entry titled "You Can Draw, and Probably Better than I Can," Roger Ebert paraphrased therapist Annette Goodheart as saying, "What you draw is an invaluable and unique representation of how you saw at that moment in that place according to your abilities. That's all we want. We already know what a dog really looks like."[6]

First- and second-year medical students in my Drawing Medicine seminar at Northwestern consistently demonstrate the power of the simple act of drawing a self-portrait in crayons. As they present their work to the rest of the class, much is revealed about the experience of being a medical student. They have drawn themselves under piles of books, or with a giant head disconnected from their body, or literally being torn between two identities—one doctor, one not. (Being a medical student is hard!) They have also drawn their hopes for their future selves as doctors, or images representing why they chose to become a doctor, or just what they miss from home.

Mind you, I don't ask for any of this. I just ask for a self-portrait in crayons. It seems from this exercise, and the ones that follow, that medical students are quite eager to explore all that they are facing via this accessible visual realm. To be clear, this is not art therapy. It is image making that may, indeed, be therapeutic, but that is not the goal. As Rita Charon describes the reflective writing her medical students do in what she calls "parallel charts," "Although I firmly believe that students derive emotional benefits from their writing . . . their emotional well-being is not the Parallel Chart's primary goal. Instead, the goals are to enable them to recognize more fully what their patients endure and to examine explicitly their own journeys through medicine."[7] Based on my experiences in teaching Drawing Medicine seminars to first- and second-year medical students and giving workshops to healthcare professionals, it is my contention that reflective drawing in professional health education can meet the same goals and be as valuable a tool as reflective writing.

Part 3: The Single Panel

In the next exercise with my medical students, I ask them to "draw the clinical encounter." Once again, the prompt is intentionally simple and vague. One student drew something like figure 6.3. When we reflected on this drawing as a class, the student who drew it said that it was in drawing this that he realized both he and the patient start a clinical encounter wondering the same thing. I pointed

fig. 6.3
MK Czerwiec, *What's Wrong?*, 2012.

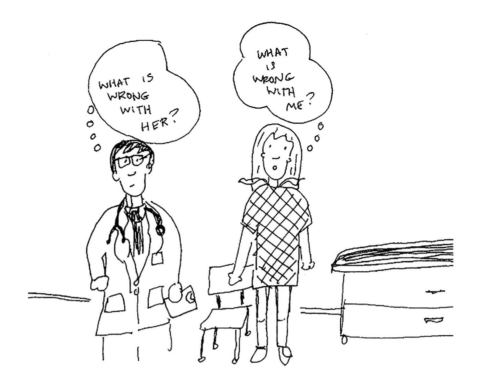

out that he drew the patient and the doctor at about the same eye level, reflecting that equality. Another student drew the doctor, the patient, and an enormous elephant. "That's what we both know but neither of us wants to talk about," she said, adding, "the elephant in the room is the fact that I have no idea what I'm doing." Another student drew a patient's hands: "It's all I can focus on. I'm too nervous to look them in the eyes. I'm working on it. But I always notice my patient's hands." One last example: a student drew the closed door to her patient's examination room. She said, "It's hard for me to see past that door. I'm so anxious. Grasping that doorknob, turning it, and opening the door is the worst part."

Through the visual nature of this exercise, we are able to reflect on the multiple perspectives available to students—as outside observer, as patient, as medical practitioner, as family present to the encounter. Students frequently report that it wasn't until being asked to draw the visual information that resonates for them in a clinical encounter that they realized what the dominant factors, barriers, and/or metaphors in those encounters are for them. They report that this exercise is enlightening as they continue to perform in their new role of doctor-in-training.

In the next set of exercises, I try to explore the students' discomfort in the state of doctor-but-not-yet-doctor by having them alternate perspectives, drawing the experience of receiving a diagnosis as a patient and then the experience of giving a diagnosis as a doctor. Students have also drawn a "mattering map"[8] of the hospital from the perspective of the medical student, and from that of the patient, noting differences and similarities. These exercises, like the others, have triggered discussions and critical moments of empathy and insight that, students report, help them think differently about what they have been doing with patients and what they might do differently moving forward.

Part 4: Making Comics

By this point in the Drawing Medicine seminar, students have developed a comfort level with their visual language, and we move on to making multipanel comics. We start by making a "jam comic,"[9] which is always great fun. As Susan Squier described earlier in this book, jam comics, loosely based on the surrealist Exquisite Corpse parlor game, involve one person drawing a comic panel and then passing it to the next person to draw the next panel. We do this for nine panels and hope for a cohesive story. The resulting comics my medical students create never fail to surprise us with their insights and humor. Like the self-portrait, this exercise serves the purpose of empowerment. The students understand from the jam comics that they already possess all the skills they need to make comics.

We then move on to making our own multipanel comics. I approach this by using Lynda Barry's "walking around an image" writing exercise.[10] The exercise involves a meditative and expository exploration of the most vivid image that comes to mind when I say the word "hospital." The homework for that week is to convert the in-class writing into a comic. Barry's writing exercise (as opposed to a more direct comic-making exercise) is intentional here. Barry has written and talked much in recent years about the important, but often overlooked, role of the image world in our lives, linking that image world to neurologic function and psychological health. She said in a 2011 interview with *The Paris Review*,

> The fastest way I can explain it is that there is this brilliant neuroscientist named V. S. Ramachandran, who wrote a book called *Phantoms in the Brain*. He was very interested in people with phantom-limb pain, and he had one patient who had lost his hand from the wrist down, but the guy's sensation was not only that the hand was still there, but that it was in a painful fist that kept clenching. Ramachandran built a box, with a mirror and two holes in one side. When the guy put his arms in, he saw the one hand reflected. When he opened the hand, he *saw* it open and it was like the missing hand was unclenching. It fixed his phantom-limb sensation. That's what I think images do; that's what the arts do. In the course of human life we have a million phantom-limb pains—losing a parent when you're little, being in a war, even something as dumb as having a mean

teacher—and seeing it somehow reflected, whether it's in our own work or listening to a song, is a way to deal with it. The Greeks knew about it. They called it catharsis, right? And without it we're fucked. I think this is the thing that keeps our mental health or emotional health in balance, and we're born with an impulse toward it.[11]

The comics the students present in class the following week often reflect this kind of "unclenching." I am using one recently submitted comic as an example (fig. 6.4), though there are many fantastic examples from the students that I could share. Kathryn spent the summer between her first and second years of medical school on a research project in Uganda. In her writing and comic-making exercise, she explored her images of the Ugandan hospital where she worked. What emerged most vividly were powerful images of these enormous, vulture-like birds that sat in massive numbers on and around the hospital. As she writes, she learned that these birds are called Marabou storks. In the next panel, she expresses her rage to a stork in the comic: "You just stand at the hospital edge, lurking, watching, contributing nothing in the midst of so many sick people." In the next panel, she realized these birds irritated her because she was projecting her own frustrations as a medical student. She closes with, "Ugh. I'm a Marabou stork." Describing this comic to the class, she said, "It wasn't until I went to draw this comic that I realized why these birds bugged me so much. In the clinic rooms with patients, I'm the Marabou stork. My research was about observation and recording, not about action or immediate change. So, I, too, stood 'lurking' in the clinic rooms with patients as a 'Marabou stork.' I don't like not being able to help when people are so sick."

Kathryn's work demonstrates what Ivan Brunetti writes in his 2011 book, *Cartooning: Philosophy and Practice*: "the deepest realizations come to us from the daily practice of drawing."[12] Brunetti also quotes cartoonist Chris Ware speaking about Ware's book *Jimmy Corrigan: The Smartest Kid on Earth*: "It developed organically as I worked on it. . . . I believe that allowing one's drawings to suggest the direction of a story is comics' single greatest formal advantage."[13] This is precisely the process Kathryn describes taking place in her comic. She realized the parallel between the Marabou storks and her researcher self as she drew the lines of the comic. She followed that realization through in her finished work, and reported that *it was the drawing process that took her there*. This is an example of what British psychoanalyst Marion Milner spoke of in *On Not Being Able to Paint*. She wrote of her free-association drawings, "They embodied a form of knowing that traditional education of the academic kind largely ignores."[14] James Kochalka puts it another way in *The Cute Manifesto* (fig. 6.5). In making comics, we gather our memories, story fragments, visual details, and our thoughts about them, just as Kochalka's figure gathers the leaves in the panels. Drawing and writing in boxes allows us to

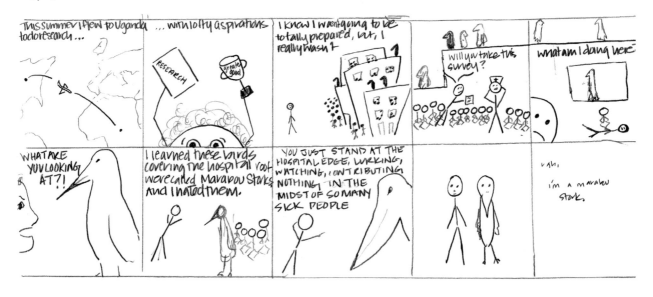

fig. 6.4
Kathryn Fay, *My Summer Vacation*, 2013.

see them together in a new way, like the leaves he throws up into the air. Wherever our memories, story fragments, visual details, and thoughts land in the finished comic, they will be different, new, and perhaps—as the comic was for my student Kathryn—revelatory.

Part 5: Beyond the Classroom

Once we have made comics together, the students and I discuss the role that making comics can play for healthcare providers in helping them be better at what they do—or even just survive.

One benefit of making comics is that it is an antidote to a work-induced condition that healthcare practitioners are at risk for, one that I call "narrative constipation."[15] Healthcare workers—nurses, doctors, therapists, chaplains, and their assistants, as well as several other high-interaction, high-stress professions, including police, fire, and emergency responders—bear witness to many profound, often gruesome, disturbing, and painful human experiences, both physical and emotional, as a matter of daily course. We are literally bombarded by images that are, ultimately, also fragments of stories. We try to process these stories and images as best we can, by discussing them with one another or perhaps, respecting the limits of HIPAA, with our loved ones. But this is inadequate, as there are so many stories unfolding day after day, and our loved ones can only hear so much.

Many of the stories are traumatic and have painful resolutions, or are left without resolution entirely. At some point, we risk just stuffing these stories, or

fig. 6.5
From James Kochalka, *The Cute Manifesto* (Gainesville, FL: Alternative Comics, 2005).

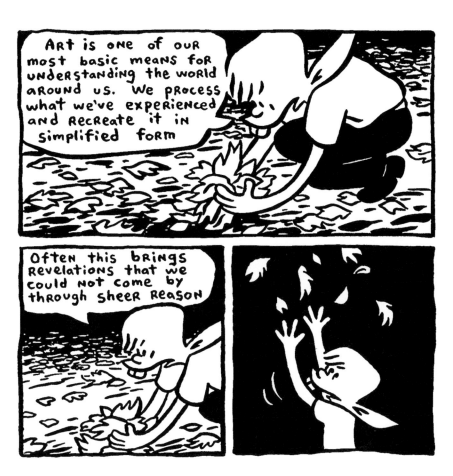

story fragments, down into our psyches to be dealt with at some later date. After all, we need to do our work. We need to be present to the patient who sits (or lies) before us. If we keep stuffing, though, these stories can affect us. One or two will almost certainly haunt us, sometimes emerging at inappropriate times and venues.

I have found the comic medium, with its simplicity and efficiency of form, to be an excellent way to process some of the more difficult stories. The comic I create about a difficult story (and my reactions to it) may not necessarily be a comic I want to share with others or publish in a book, but it is something that helps keep me regular. I can draw a simple four- or eight-panel comic in my daily sketchbook, and I am able to get those images out of my head, onto paper, where I try to weave them into a larger narrative, integrating what I've witnessed into my stories. Then I can choose to either hold on to them or let them go. This drawing equips me to continue as an effective caregiver. The payoff is enormous and essential. Its value, I can attest, is found not only in professional caregiving but also in caregiving for family members and, as several graphic novels attest, in living with a challenging illness.

Another benefit of comic making is as a way to parse out the elements and narratives of a bioethical dilemma. Such dilemmas, by their nature, can easily be overwhelming and complex. The sequential box (or implied box) structure of a comic can provide a kind of safe and quiet place to examine a larger situation—one box, one moment, one element, at a time. For a terrific example of this in action, see my co-author Michael Green's comic *Missed It*, published in the *Annals of Internal Medicine* in March 2013, which describes a medical mistake that resulted in a patient's death.[16] In the comic, Green describes a situation from his residency that has haunted him for years.

> The incident itself was so unsettling that I needed to find a way to reach a resolution about the events of that evening. I drafted a raw and urgent short story, and this helped me release many of the feelings that I had been holding inside for so long. But ultimately, I felt that the story required more than just words—that it also required images to depict the intensity of the emotions of that night. In creating the comic I was able to shape and define not only what happened, but also the meaning of those events. While I'm no longer haunted by this patient's death, the comic gives substance to my experience and helps frame the way I understand what transpired.[17]

The comic has unexpectedly proven to be a useful teaching tool. He writes,

> Since publishing "Missed It," I have used the comic as a teaching tool on several occasions. The physicians with whom I've shared the story clearly relate with the main character, and this helps the story serve as an effective springboard for discussion about their own anxieties and fears about making a medical mistake. This then segues into a discussion of structural contributions to medical mistakes, and how errors might be avoided by, for example, restructuring on-call schedules, changing how doctors are supervised at night, and improving communication between healthcare teams. In short the comic has been a valuable resource for teaching about important topics related to professionalism in medicine.[18]

Yet another benefit of comic making is that it keeps creative skills, so critical to diagnosis and treatment, sharp. In a commentary in *Academic Medicine*, author Niamh Kelly states, "When encouraged and allowed to flourish, creativity, with its hallmark features of imaginative thinking linked with the spirit of inquiry, has been and will continue to be responsible for continuous breakthroughs in the practice of medicine."[19] Kelly closes the essay by encouraging physicians to ask one another, "What are you doing creatively these days?"[20] I

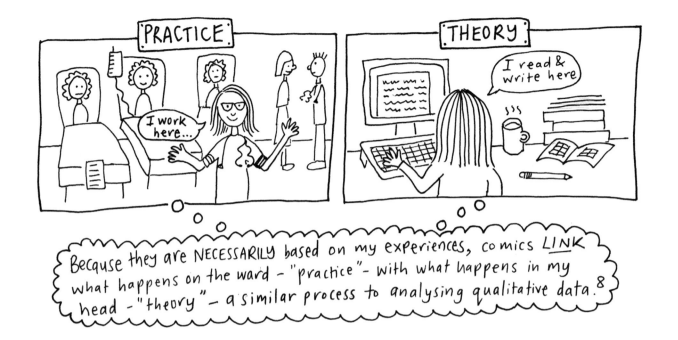

fig. 6.6
Muna Al-Jawad, *Bridging Practice and Theory*, 2012.

think "Making comics!" would be a fantastic answer, one likely to lead to very creative conversations.

One last example of the benefit of comic making in medicine can be seen in the work of geriatrician Muna Al-Jawad, who is studying, as she describes it, "how people learn to be geriatricians."[21] Figure 6.6 is an excerpt from her comic, published in the *Journal of Medical Humanities* as "Comics Are Research: Graphic Narratives as a New Way of Seeing Clinical Practice."[22] Al-Jawad proposes that making comics links practice and theory.

In an interview for this piece, Al-Jawad said,

> In my ethnographic research, I was struggling to write about my feelings, but when I drew the comic I was able to access that easily. I found myself really angry about one situation. It all came out doing the comic. I thought, "Maybe there is something here." Comics are a way to get to my feelings, a way that doesn't come across sloppy or cheesy. With comics you can do multiple things—narrative thread, image, speech, thoughts—all in one picture. Comics allow you to see under the surface of situations and narratives in a kind of shorthand.[23]

These examples demonstrate the value of making comics in the practice of medicine, far beyond the classroom. It is my hope that these are merely early examples, and more will emerge as the use of reflective drawing gains respect and use in medicine.

Conclusion

Though I love each session of my Drawing Medicine seminar, our last meeting is often my favorite. For this final session, students read and present to their classmates a work of graphic medicine—that is, an existing graphic novel with medical content. It would be fantastic if the students and I could all read and discuss the same graphic medicine text in this course, but we only have five weeks, much of which we spend drawing, and I want to expose the students to as many of the comics on medical themes as I can. So each of them chooses one book-length comic on a medical theme to read and present to the class. But I put a twist on the final assignment. They have to do a third-grade-style book report, one that includes presenting their books to us in a visual form. Here again, I leave the directive vague, to see where they take the assignment. My goal is to have them use these illness narratives presented in visual form as a bridge toward using reflective drawing to respond to stories of suffering and loss as they move forward in their medical careers. In using this "third-grade" approach, my hope is that they learn to engage with the story on its own visual terms with their unique visual languages. This culmination of our five-week course aims to equip students with a tool, again paraphrasing Rita Charon, to use in recognizing more fully what our patients endure and examining explicitly their own journeys through healthcare.[24]

One student made a poster of cut-out breasts from magazine ads in response to Marissa Marchetto's *Cancer Vixen*. In describing her poster, she discussed how *Cancer Vixen* caused her to revisit representations of women in popular media, and her act of cutting the breasts out of advertisements was reminiscent, for her, of Marchetto's visual imagery of the biopsy scalpel and the looming threat of breast removal due to the cancer. One student showed a StoryCorps cartoon in response to Brian Fies's *Mom's Cancer*. One student mounted the drawn pages of her report on multicolored sheets of construction paper and tied them together with yarn. One student, mirroring the themes of Nate Powell's *Swallow Me Whole*, colored layers and layers of crayons, topped those with a field of solid black, and then, using a toothpick, he "carved" his drawing of a frog. Students have redrawn the characters from David Small's *Stitches*, Sarah Leavitt's *Tangles*, and Charles Burns's *Black Hole*, as well as single images that represent thematic aspects of Darryl Cunningham's *Psychiatric Tales* and Joyce Farmer's *Special Exits*. Whatever they do, it is always amazing to watch: in five weeks the students have begun to reclaim a bit of what they may have left behind when they, perhaps, were chosen as the students who would excel in math or science, when they were encouraged to stop drawing and "get serious." They now remember anew that they can draw, that we all can. They have laid claim to their drawings and to their individual styles. These future doctors have come to understand that drawing—even with crayons—in the service of their ideas and experiences, as reflection or as its own reward, *is* serious.

· · · · · · · · ·

The comic excerpts that follow—from Miriam Engelberg's *Cancer Made Me a Shallower Person: A Memoir in Comics* and geriatrician Muna Al-Jawad's Tumblr, *Old Person Whisperer*—bear witness to some of the benefits derived from making and reading comics in the healthcare context. Their simplicity in style is belied by the power of their content.

FIGURES ON
FOLLOWING PAGES
▬ ▬ ▬ ▬ ▬ ▬

fig. 6.7

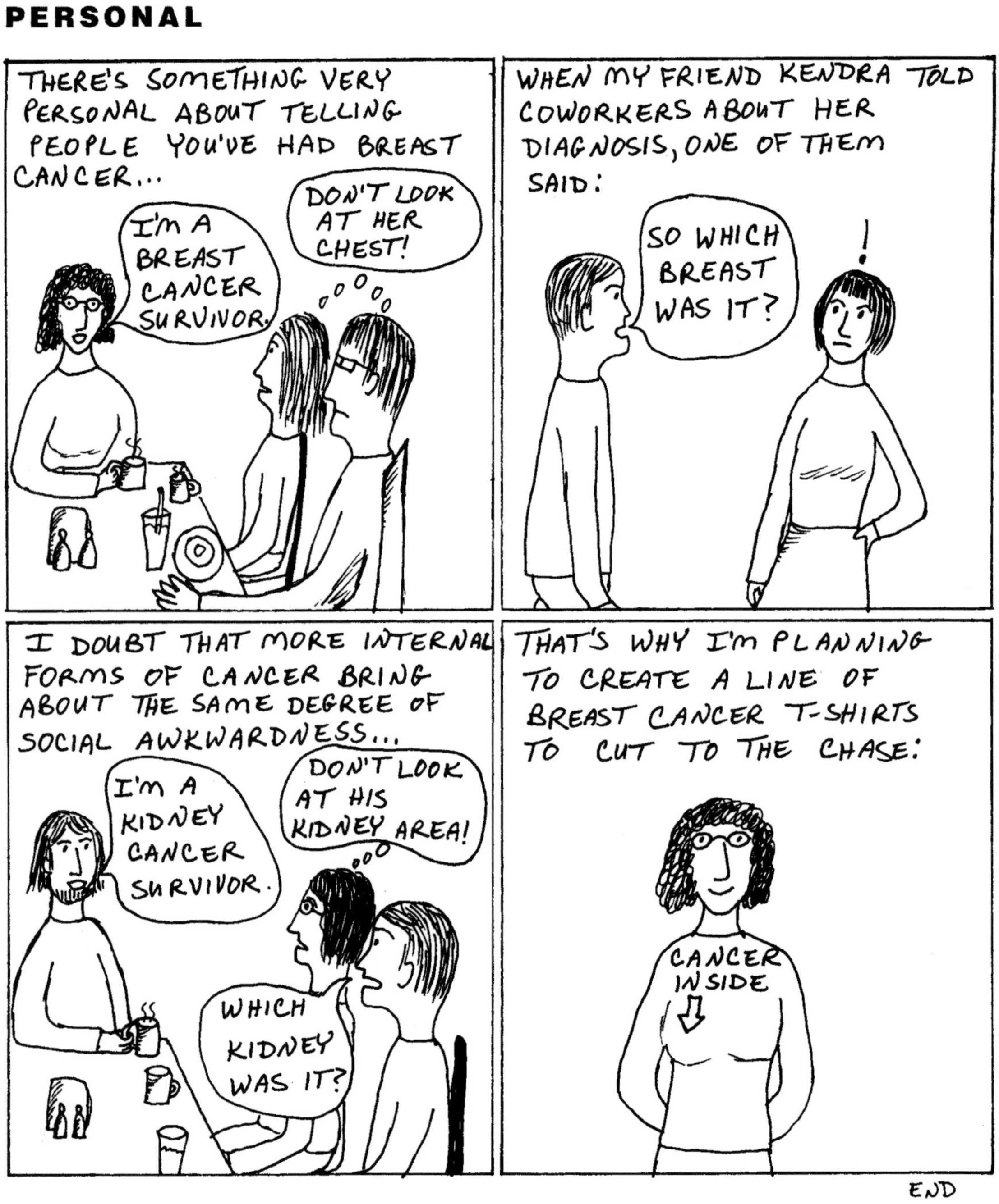
PERSONAL
THERE'S SOMETHING VERY PERSONAL ABOUT TELLING PEOPLE YOU'VE HAD BREAST CANCER...
I'M A BREAST CANCER SURVIVOR.
DON'T LOOK AT HER CHEST!
WHEN MY FRIEND KENDRA TOLD COWORKERS ABOUT HER DIAGNOSIS, ONE OF THEM SAID:
SO WHICH BREAST WAS IT?
!
I DOUBT THAT MORE INTERNAL FORMS OF CANCER BRING ABOUT THE SAME DEGREE OF SOCIAL AWKWARDNESS...
I'M A KIDNEY CANCER SURVIVOR.
DON'T LOOK AT HIS KIDNEY AREA!
WHICH KIDNEY WAS IT?
THAT'S WHY I'M PLANNING TO CREATE A LINE OF BREAST CANCER T-SHIRTS TO CUT TO THE CHASE:
CANCER INSIDE
END

fig. 6.8

SPIRITUALITY

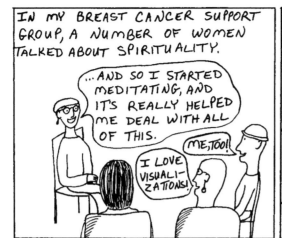

IN MY BREAST CANCER SUPPORT GROUP, A NUMBER OF WOMEN TALKED ABOUT SPIRITUALITY.

...AND SO I STARTED MEDITATING, AND IT'S REALLY HELPED ME DEAL WITH ALL OF THIS.

ME, TOO!

I LOVE VISUALIZATIONS!

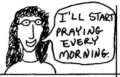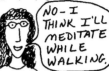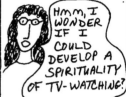

EVEN BEFORE MY DIAGNOSIS I'D BEEN TRYING TO DEVELOP SOME SORT OF SPIRITUAL PRACTICE...

I'LL START PRAYING EVERY MORNING.

NO—I THINK I'LL MEDITATE WHILE WALKING.

MAYBE WRITING IN A SPIRITUAL JOURNAL WOULD WORK BETTER FOR ME.

HMM, I WONDER IF I COULD DEVELOP A SPIRITUALITY OF TV-WATCHING?

AND NOW HERE I WAS FACING A SERIOUS ILLNESS, AND INSTEAD OF FINDING INNER STRENGTH I WAS GOING IN THE OPPOSITE DIRECTION.

HONEY, WHAT WAS THE NAME OF THE HOST OF "LET'S MAKE A DEAL"? 9 LETTERS.

...WHICH WAS ODD CONSIDERING MY BACKGROUND...

I HAVE A MASTER'S DEGREE IN THEOLOGY! I USED TO DO CENTERING PRAYER TWICE A DAY, FOR GOD'S SAKE!

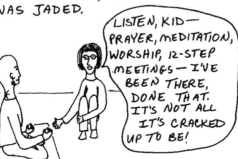

THAT'S WHEN I REALIZED I'D DONE IT ALL BACKWARD; I'D HAD MY SPIRITUAL ADVENTURES IN MY YOUTH, AND NOW I WAS JADED.

LISTEN, KID— PRAYER, MEDITATION, WORSHIP, 12-STEP MEETINGS—I'VE BEEN THERE, DONE THAT. IT'S NOT ALL IT'S CRACKED UP TO BE!

I KNOW IT SEEMS FUN AND EXCITING RIGHT NOW, BUT THINK OF YOUR FUTURE! SOMEDAY YOU'LL NEED A SPIRITUAL AWAKENING... DON'T USE IT UP TOO SOON!

fig. 6.9

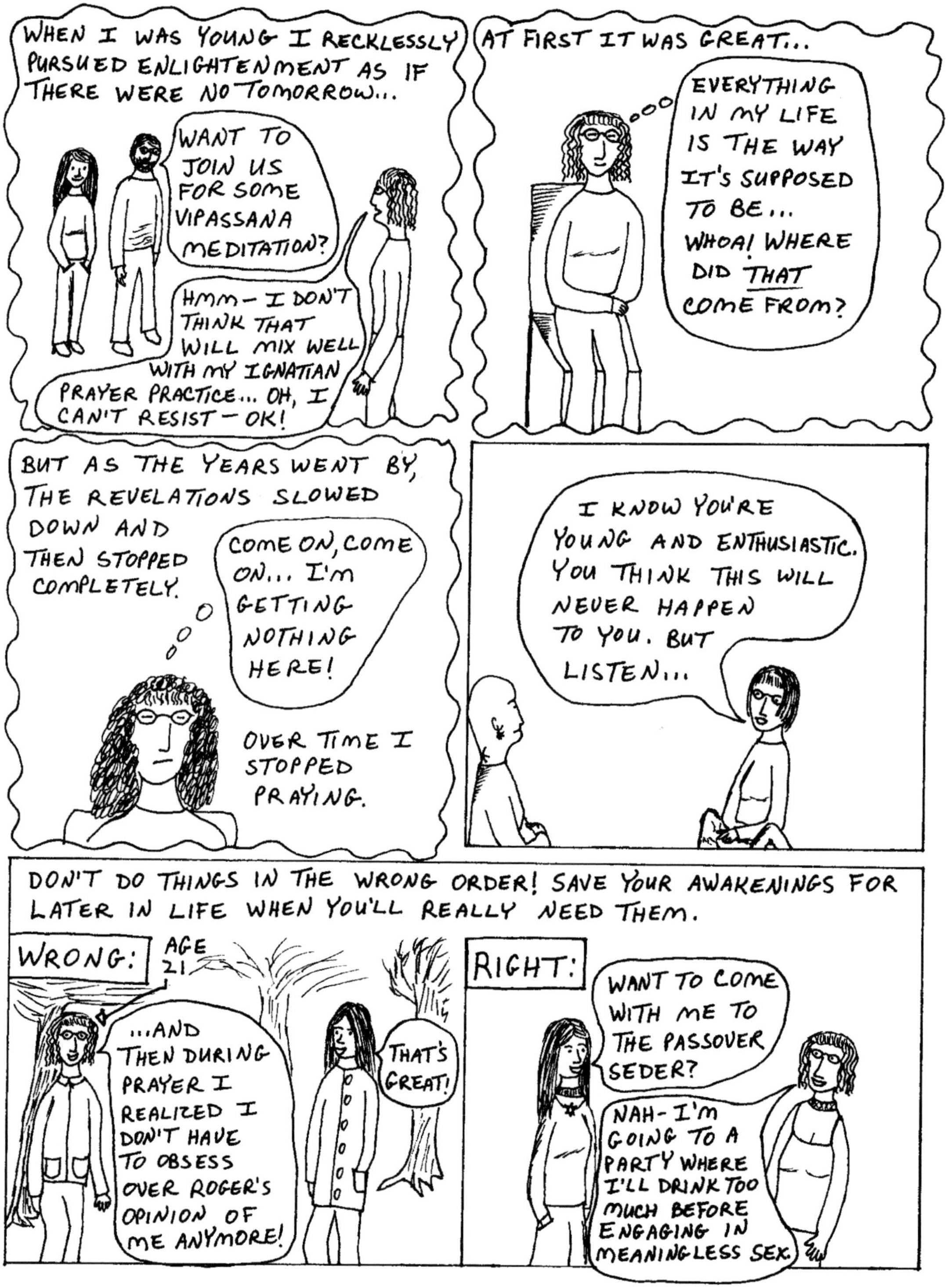

WHEN I WAS YOUNG I RECKLESSLY PURSUED ENLIGHTENMENT AS IF THERE WERE NO TOMORROW...
WANT TO JOIN US FOR SOME VIPASSANA MEDITATION?
HMM– I DON'T THINK THAT WILL MIX WELL WITH MY IGNATIAN PRAYER PRACTICE... OH, I CAN'T RESIST– OK!
AT FIRST IT WAS GREAT...
EVERYTHING IN MY LIFE IS THE WAY IT'S SUPPOSED TO BE... WHOA! WHERE DID THAT COME FROM?
BUT AS THE YEARS WENT BY, THE REVELATIONS SLOWED DOWN AND THEN STOPPED COMPLETELY.
COME ON, COME ON... I'M GETTING NOTHING HERE!
OVER TIME I STOPPED PRAYING.
I KNOW YOU'RE YOUNG AND ENTHUSIASTIC. YOU THINK THIS WILL NEVER HAPPEN TO YOU. BUT LISTEN...
DON'T DO THINGS IN THE WRONG ORDER! SAVE YOUR AWAKENINGS FOR LATER IN LIFE WHEN YOU'LL REALLY NEED THEM.
WRONG:
AGE 21
...AND THEN DURING PRAYER I REALIZED I DON'T HAVE TO OBSESS OVER ROGER'S OPINION OF ME ANYMORE!
THAT'S GREAT!
RIGHT:
WANT TO COME WITH ME TO THE PASSOVER SEDER?
NAH– I'M GOING TO A PARTY WHERE I'LL DRINK TOO MUCH BEFORE ENGAGING IN MEANINGLESS SEX.

fig. 6.10

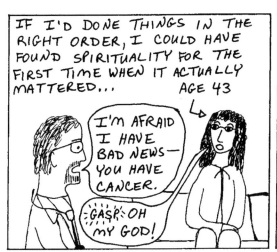

IF I'D DONE THINGS IN THE RIGHT ORDER, I COULD HAVE FOUND SPIRITUALITY FOR THE FIRST TIME WHEN IT ACTUALLY MATTERED...   AGE 43

I'M AFRAID I HAVE BAD NEWS— YOU HAVE CANCER.

GASP! OH MY GOD!

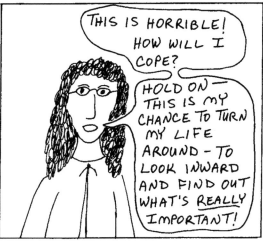

THIS IS HORRIBLE! HOW WILL I COPE?

HOLD ON— THIS IS MY CHANCE TO TURN MY LIFE AROUND — TO LOOK INWARD AND FIND OUT WHAT'S REALLY IMPORTANT!

BUT NO — IT WAS TOO LATE FOR THAT. SPIRITUAL BREAKTHROUGHS ARE LIKE CHEMO—YOU CAN'T GO BACK TO A TYPE YOU'VE HAD BEFORE.

IT DOESN'T MATTER WHAT ROGER THINKS OF YOU...

ROGER? THAT BOYFRIEND FROM 1979?! WHO CARES? I NEED HELP FACING MY MORTALITY HERE!

I DID, HOWEVER, HAVE A REVELATION DURING CHEMO...

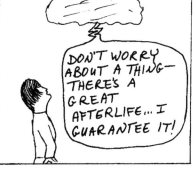

DON'T WORRY ABOUT A THING— THERE'S A GREAT AFTERLIFE... I GUARANTEE IT!

NO, NOT THAT KIND OF REVELATION—THIS KIND...

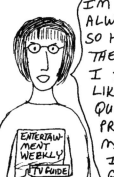

I'M SICK OF ALWAYS TRYING SO HARD TO DO THE RIGHT THING. I DON'T FEEL LIKE SITTING QUIETLY AND PRAYING OR MEDITATING, SO I'M NOT GONNA!

ENTERTAINMENT WEEKLY
TV GUIDE

AND THEN I HEARD A TALK AT THE HOSPITAL...

WHEN I WAS FIRST DIAGNOSED I CONSIDERED TAKING UP YOGA OR MEDITATION AS MY SPIRITUAL PRACTICE, BUT I ENDED UP DECIDING ON MUSIC.

fig. 6.11

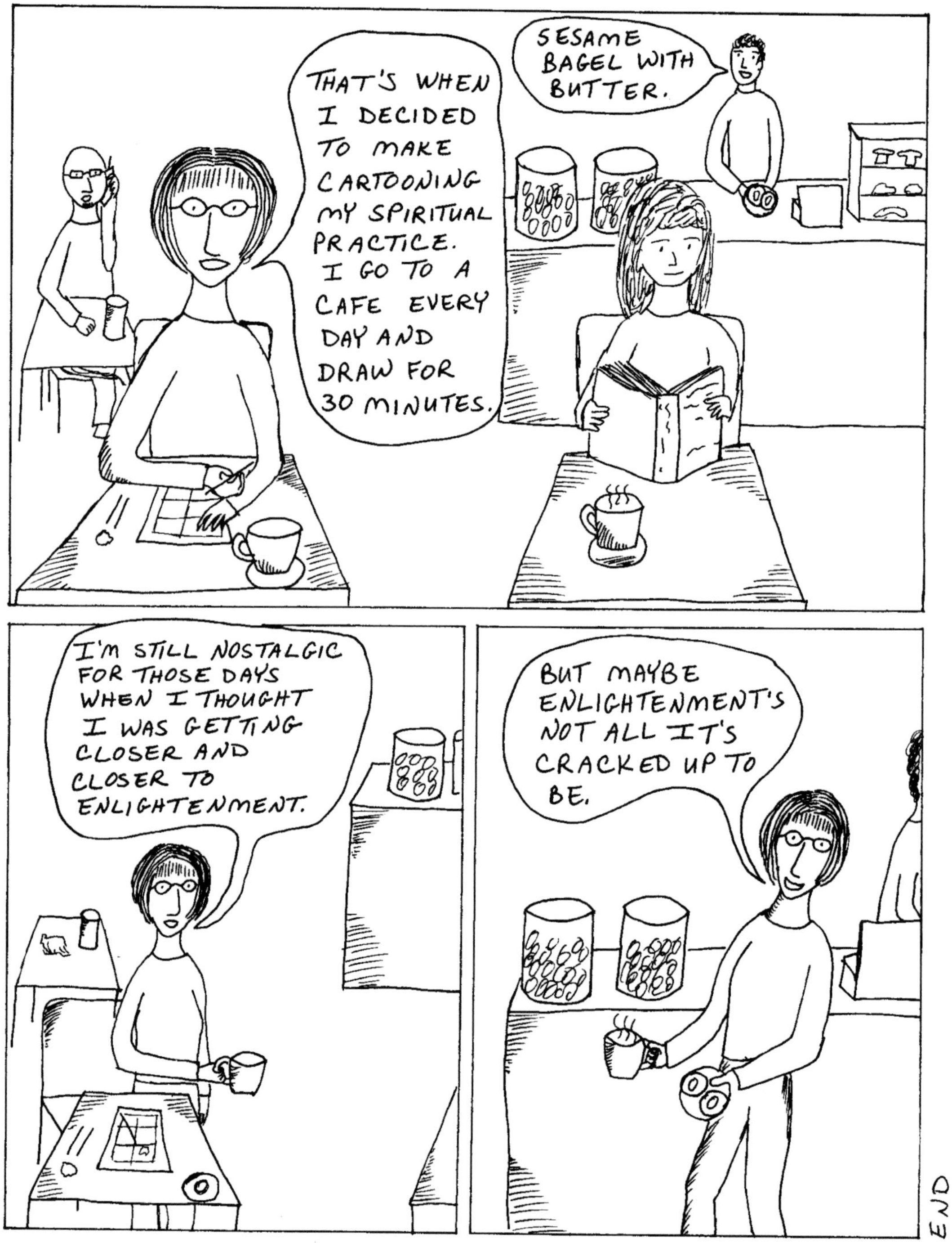
THAT'S WHEN I DECIDED TO MAKE CARTOONING MY SPIRITUAL PRACTICE. I GO TO A CAFE EVERY DAY AND DRAW FOR 30 MINUTES.
SESAME BAGEL WITH BUTTER.
I'M STILL NOSTALGIC FOR THOSE DAYS WHEN I THOUGHT I WAS GETTING CLOSER AND CLOSER TO ENLIGHTENMENT.
BUT MAYBE ENLIGHTENMENT'S NOT ALL IT'S CRACKED UP TO BE.
END

fig. 6.12

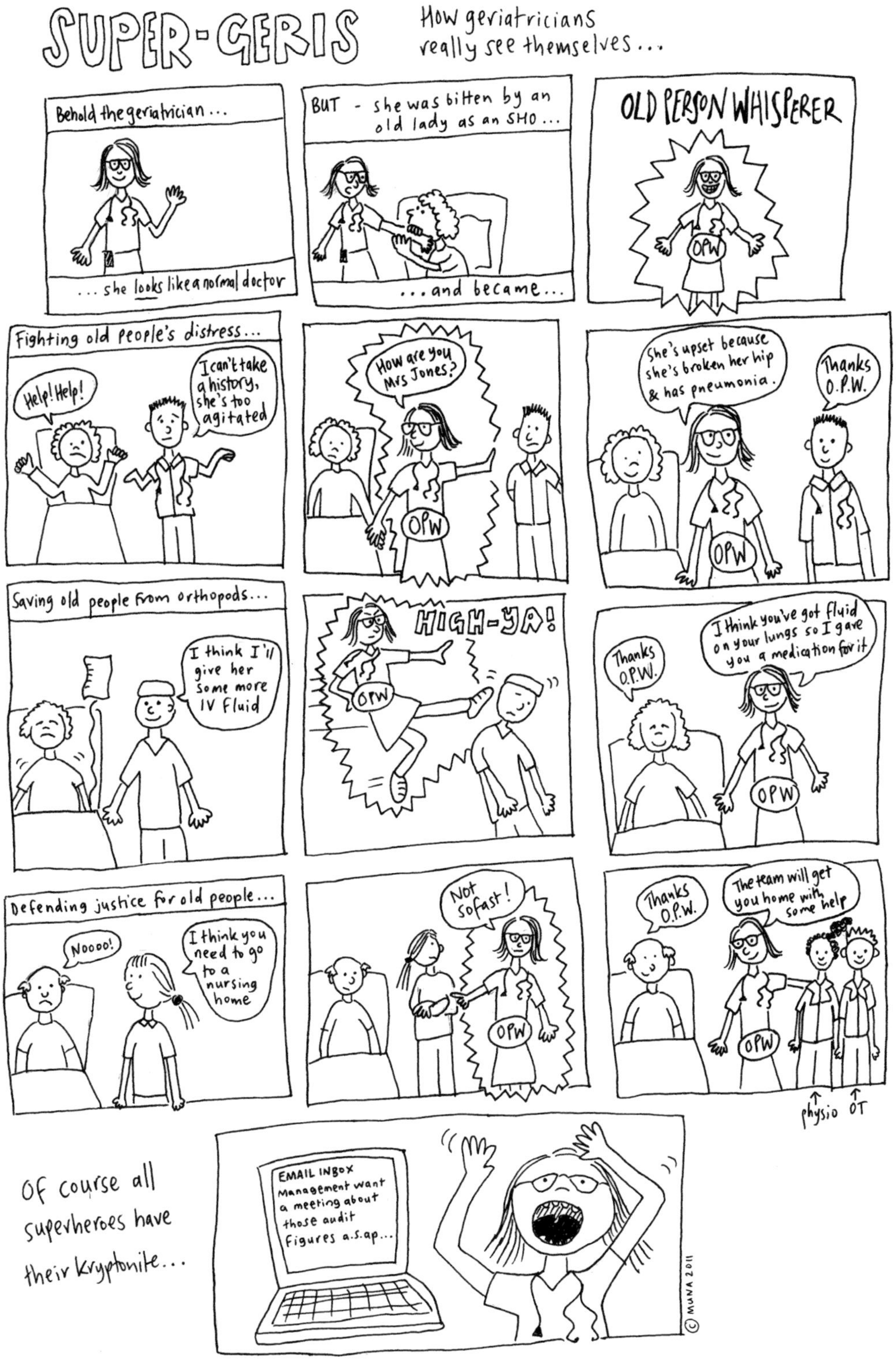
SUPER-GERIS
How geriatricians really see themselves...
Behold the geriatrician...
... she looks like a normal doctor
BUT - she was bitten by an old lady as an SHO...
...and became...
OLD PERSON WHISPERER
OPW
Fighting old people's distress...
Help! Help!
I can't take a history, she's too agitated
How are you Mrs Jones?
OPW
She's upset because she's broken her hip & has pneumonia.
Thanks O.P.W.
OPW
Saving old people from orthopods...
I think I'll give her some more IV Fluid
HIGH-YA!
OPW
Thanks O.P.W.
I think you've got fluid on your lungs so I gave you a medication for it.
OPW
Defending justice for old people...
Noooo!
I think you need to go to a nursing home
Not so fast!
OPW
Thanks O.P.W.
The team will get you home with some help
OPW
physio
OT
Of course all superheroes have their kryptonite...
EMAIL INBOX
Management want a meeting about those audit figures a.s.ap...
© MUNA 2011

Conclusion

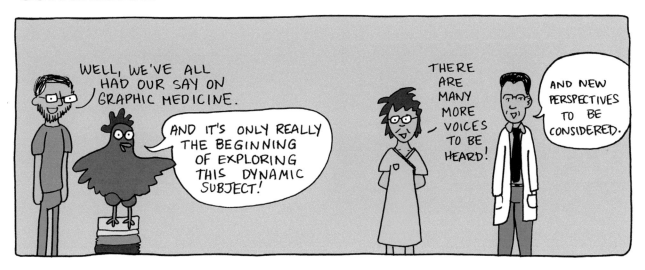

WELL, WE'VE ALL HAD OUR SAY ON GRAPHIC MEDICINE.

AND IT'S ONLY REALLY THE BEGINNING OF EXPLORING THIS DYNAMIC SUBJECT!

THERE ARE MANY MORE VOICES TO BE HEARD!

AND NEW PERSPECTIVES TO BE CONSIDERED.

HERE'S AN IDEA! LET'S ASK A FEW PEOPLE WHO HAVE COME TO COMICS AND MEDICINE CONFERENCES OR CONTACTED US THROUGH THE GRAPHIC MEDICINE WEBSITE TO SHARE WHAT GRAPHIC MEDICINE MEANS TO THEM!

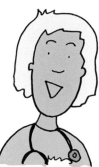

NOT A BAD IDEA, MK. PERHAPS FROM THEM WE WILL CONVEY A SENSE OF THE COMMUNITY THAT HAS FORMED AT THE INTERSECTION OF COMICS AND MEDICINE...

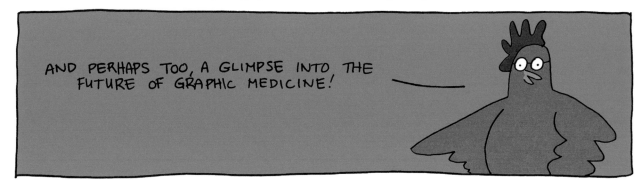

AND PERHAPS TOO, A GLIMPSE INTO THE FUTURE OF GRAPHIC MEDICINE!

Alex Thomas & Gary Ashwal

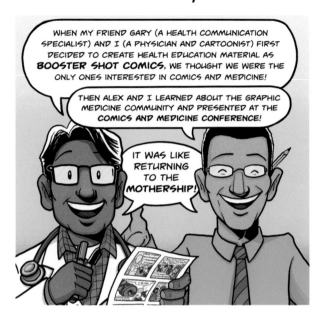

WHEN MY FRIEND GARY (A HEALTH COMMUNICATION SPECIALIST) AND I (A PHYSICIAN AND CARTOONIST) FIRST DECIDED TO CREATE HEALTH EDUCATION MATERIAL AS **BOOSTER SHOT COMICS**, WE THOUGHT WE WERE THE ONLY ONES INTERESTED IN COMICS AND MEDICINE!

THEN ALEX AND I LEARNED ABOUT THE GRAPHIC MEDICINE COMMUNITY AND PRESENTED AT THE COMICS AND MEDICINE CONFERENCE!

IT WAS LIKE RETURNING TO THE **MOTHERSHIP!**

Rinko Endo

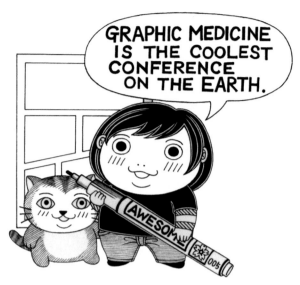

GRAPHIC MEDICINE IS THE COOLEST CONFERENCE ON THE EARTH.

Mat Defiler

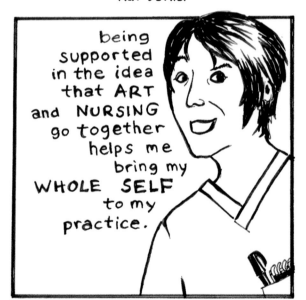

being supported in the idea that ART and NURSING go together helps me bring my WHOLE SELF to my practice.

Joyce Farmer

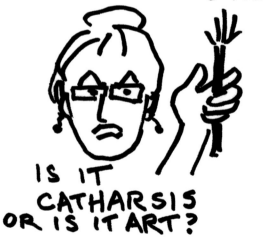

GRAPHIC MEDICINE:

IS IT CATHARSIS OR IS IT ART?

Andrew Godfrey

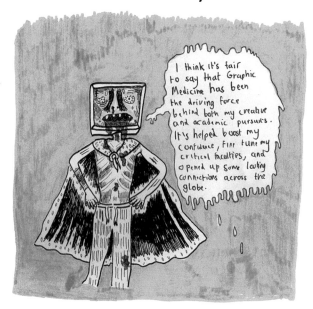

I think it's fair to say that Graphic Medicine has been the driving force behind both my creative and academic pursuits. It's helped boost my confidence, fine tune my critical faculties, and opened up some lasting connections across the globe.

Katie Green

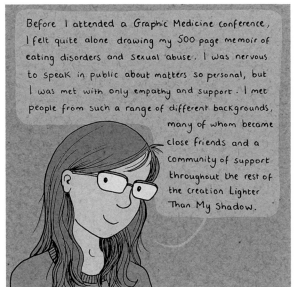

Before I attended a Graphic Medicine conference, I felt quite alone, drawing my 500 page memoir of eating disorders and sexual abuse. I was nervous to speak in public about matters so personal, but I was met with only empathy and support. I met people from such a range of different backgrounds, many of whom became close friends and a community of support throughout the rest of the creation Lighter Than My Shadow.

Lydia Gregg

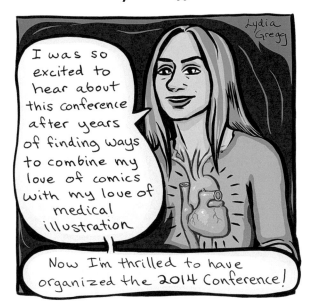

I was so excited to hear about this conference after years of finding ways to combine my love of comics with my love of medical illustration

Now I'm thrilled to have organized the 2014 Conference!

Michelle Huang

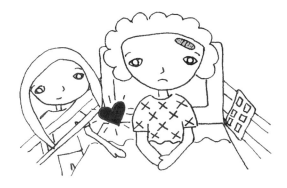

MY MOTHER HAD A STROKE WHEN I WAS ELEVEN.

FOR CAREGIVERS, GRAPHIC MEDICINE PROVIDES A VISUAL LANGUAGE TO REPRESENT THE SILENT MOMENTS OF AFFECTIVE CONNECTION LEFT UNACKNOWLEDGED BY MEDICAL DISCOURSE.

Paula Knight

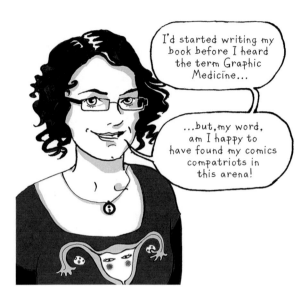

I'd started writing my book before I heard the term Graphic Medicine...

...but, my word, am I happy to have found my comics compatriots in this arena!

Cathy Leamy

MY FAVORITE MOMENTS COME RIGHT AFTER I SHOW STAFF MEMBERS AT MY HOSPITAL WHY COMICS WORK SO WELL FOR HEALTHCARE COMMUNICATION.

YOU CAN JUST SEE SPARKS GO OFF IN THEIR HEADS, AND THEY BUBBLE UP SO MANY IDEAS!

HUH, I BET WE COULD USE COMICS TO EXPLAIN PROCEDURES TO LOW-LITERACY PATIENTS!

YUP!

OUR ONLINE TRAINING MODULES ARE BORING. WHAT IF WE MADE A WEBCOMIC INSTEAD?

LET'S TRY IT!

Sarah Leavitt

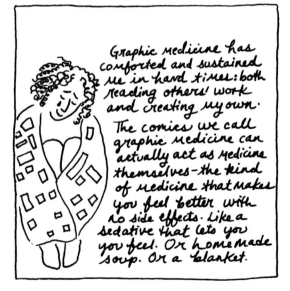

Graphic medicine has comforted and sustained me in hard times: both reading others' work and creating my own.

The comics we call graphic medicine can actually act as medicine themselves - the kind of medicine that makes you feel better with no side effects. Like a sedative that lets you you feel. Or homemade soup. Or a blanket.

Sarah Lightman

AN ALPHABET ART HERSTORY OF MEDICINE—

C is for colic and crying ~~baby~~ mother

26 JANUARY 2014 3am

Back from hospital My delightful newborn son hails allnight

We try Infacol.

My beautiful calm and alert son returns

GRAPHIC MEDICINE. HUMANITY IN THE HUMANITIES. PANEL BY PANEL BREAKING DOWN THE COLD DETACHED ACADEMIC WORLD PLACING A BROKEN BLEEDING HEART IN THE CENTRE.

Meredith Li-Vollmer

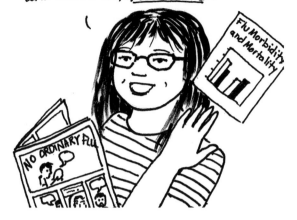

Comics help me make public health issues CONCRETE, *intimate*, accessible, and above all, *human*.

Mita Mahato

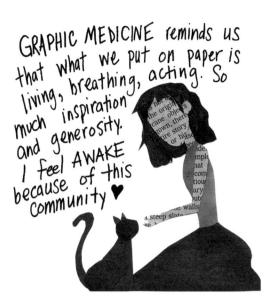

GRAPHIC MEDICINE reminds us that what we put on paper is living, breathing, acting. So much inspiration and generosity. I feel AWAKE because of this community ♥

Juliet McMullin

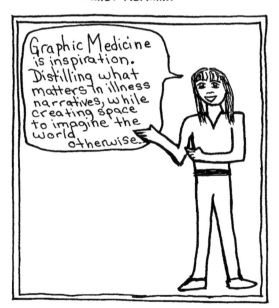

Graphic Medicine is inspiration. Distilling what matters in illness narratives, while creating space to imagine the world otherwise.

Nancy K. Miller

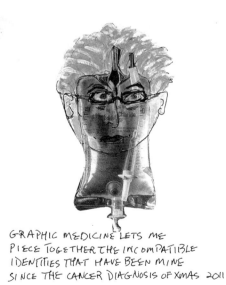

GRAPHIC MEDICINE LETS ME PIECE TOGETHER THE INCOMPATIBLE IDENTITIES THAT HAVE BEEN MINE SINCE THE CANCER DIAGNOSIS OF XMAS 2011

Ryan Montoya

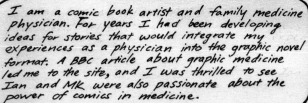

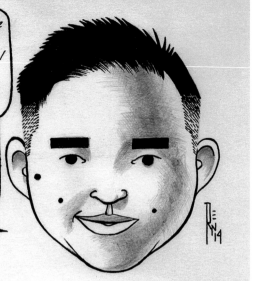

I am a comic book artist and family medicine physician. For years I had been developing ideas for stories that would integrate my experiences as a physician into the graphic novel format. A BBC article about graphic medicine led me to the site, and I was thrilled to see Ian and MK were also passionate about the power of comics in medicine.

Graphic Medicine has compelled me to think and write critically about comic books that deal with issues in medicine. Through Twitter, it has also afforded me the chance to interface directly with the creators of these works - an incredible opportunity I never would have had otherwise.

Linda Raphael

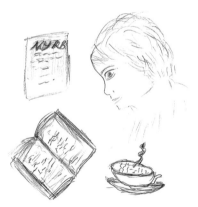

"Teaching graphic-medicine texts is novel and exciting! This remarkable genre offers new approaches to the old subject of ambiguity in human existence. The multiple, complementary, and competing storylines unique to concurrent visual and textual "telling" - often represented on a single page or in one frame - are anything but limited to one interpretation."

Theresa Rojas

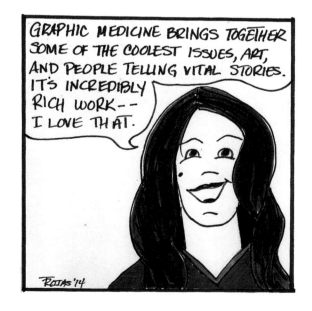

GRAPHIC MEDICINE BRINGS TOGETHER SOME OF THE COOLEST ISSUES, ART, AND PEOPLE TELLING VITAL STORIES. IT'S INCREDIBLY RICH WORK -- I LOVE THAT.

Veta Salubi

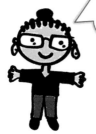

Hi, I'm Veta and I wrote the comic 'Saving Grace', a story of breast cancer survival for public awareness in my country. Without Graphic Medicine, I would not have believed that I could make a difference by merging my work and my passion- to write and showcase comic stories that make a difference. Thank you GM for the support and encouragement. I needed it.

ET Russian

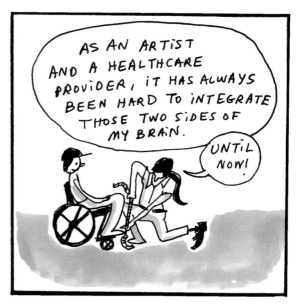

David Small

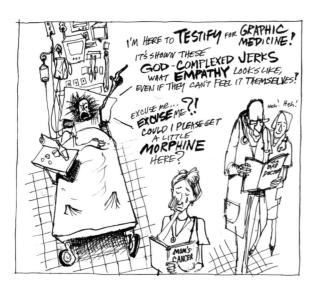

Nicola Streeten

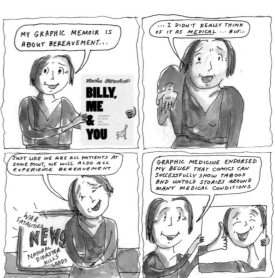

John Swogger

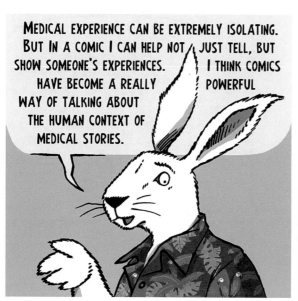

MEDICAL EXPERIENCE CAN BE EXTREMELY ISOLATING. BUT IN A COMIC I CAN HELP NOT JUST TELL, BUT SHOW SOMEONE'S EXPERIENCES. I THINK COMICS HAVE BECOME A REALLY POWERFUL WAY OF TALKING ABOUT THE HUMAN CONTEXT OF MEDICAL STORIES.

Shelly Wall

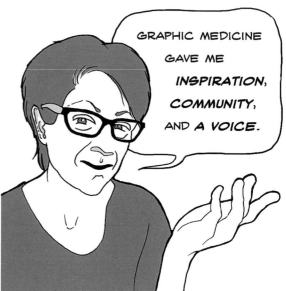

GRAPHIC MEDICINE GAVE ME *INSPIRATION*, *COMMUNITY*, AND *A VOICE*.

Amerisa Waters

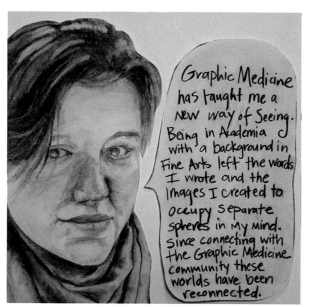

Graphic Medicine has taught me a new way of Seeing. Being in Academia with a background in Fine Arts left the words I wrote and the Images I created to occupy separate spheres in my mind. Since connecting with the Graphic Medicine community these worlds have been reconnected.

Nye Wright

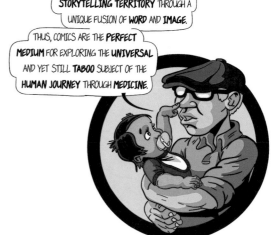

COMICS ARE **POWERFUL** BECAUSE OF THEIR ABILITY TO PROBE **UNEXPLORED STORYTELLING TERRITORY** THROUGH A UNIQUE FUSION OF **WORD** AND **IMAGE**.

THUS, COMICS ARE THE **PERFECT MEDIUM** FOR EXPLORING THE **UNIVERSAL** AND YET STILL **TABOO** SUBJECT OF THE **HUMAN JOURNEY** THROUGH **MEDICINE**.

NOTES

Chapter 1

1. For overviews of comic scholarship, see Witek, "Comics Criticism"; Chute, "Decoding Comics"; and Beaty, "In Focus," which features a series of essays dedicated to comics studies (with special attention to intersections with film studies).

2. Examples of journals include *Word & Image*; Lent, *International Journal of Comic Art*; *Image and Narrative*; Ault, *ImageText*; *European Comic Art*; *Journal of Graphic Novels and Comics*; *Studies in Comics*; and *Comics Grid*. Non-academic periodicals include Groth, *Comics Journal*; Cooke, *Comic Book Artist*; Hignite, *Comic Art*; and Eury, *Back Issue*. See also the various resources collected by Gene Kannenberg Jr. at comicsresearch.org (last updated October 1, 2010). The University Press of Mississippi (UPM) has been the leading academic publisher in comics studies to date. Jeet Heer has suggested that the UPM list effectively made comics studies into "a coherent field." See Heer, "The Rise of Comics Scholarship: The Role of the University Press of Mississippi," *Sans Everything* (blog), August 2, 2008, http://sanseverything. wordpress.com/2008/08/02 /the-rise-of-comics-scholarship-the-role-of-university-press-of-mississippi/).

3. Hatfield, "Defining Comics," 19.

4. Smith, "It Ain't Easy," 111.

5. Due to demands of space, I limit my survey mainly to books (both monographs and essay collections). This focus is not intended to slight the substantial and important work that has appeared in articles, interviews, and reviews, both in print and online.

6. Feiffer, *Great Comic Book Heroes*; Blackbeard and Williams, *Smithsonian Collection*; and Barrier and Williams, *Smithsonian Book*.

7. There was, of course, worthwhile criticism on comics prior to the 1960s. For a collection of essays written in the earlier twentieth century, see Heer and Worcester, *Arguing Comics*. See also Witek, "Comics Criticism," and Zorbaugh, "Comics as an Educational Medium," a special issue of the *Journal of Educational Sociology*.

8. See Kunzle, *Early Comic Strip* and *History of the Comic Strip*; Barker, *Haunt of Fears*; Witek, *Comic Books*. Witek's book was one of UPM's first titles in comics studies. Other social histories include Nyberg, *Seal of Approval*; Rubenstein, *Bad Language*; Wright, *Comic Book Nation*; Jones, *Men of*

Tomorrow; Beaty, *Fredric Wertham*; Gabilliet, *Of Comics*; and Hajdu, *Ten-Cent Plague*. For a history of the comics industry told in comics form, see Van Lente and Dunlavey's 2012 *The Comic Book History of Comics*, which was originally published in six individual issues as *Comic Book Comics* between 2008 and 2011.

9. *The Comics Journal* began publication in 1976 as *The New Nostalgia Journal*, changing to its current name the following year. Roger Sabin has assessed the importance of *The Comics Journal* as follows: "Under the editorship of Gary Groth, superhero and 'collecting' stories were progressively eschewed in favour of evaluative criticism of the more mature titles, coupled with a campaigning attitude to creators' rights and a scholarly approach to comics history. Although the style was often verbose, the *Journal* was in effect a new kind of fanzine, and provided much-needed proof that such publications need not be mindlessly sycophantic and uncritical" (*Adult Comics*, 85). For an in-house assessment of *The Comics Journal* and its importance for comics criticism, see Rich Kreiner, "The Firing Line Forms Here," *The Comics Journal*, posted January 1, 2010, http://classic.tcj.com/tcj-300/tcj-300-meet-the-comics-press.

10. An interesting thread from *The Comics Journal*'s message board on the formation and currency of the term "graphic novel" has been preserved at the blog *tics, tics & tics*. See Andrei Molotiu, "The Origins of the Term 'Graphic Novel'—a Thread Rescued from the Old *Comics Journal* Message Board," *tics, tics & tics* (blog), January 15, 2014, http://ticsticsandtics.blogspot.com/2014/01/the-origins-of-term-graphic-novel.html#more.

11. Sabin, *Adult Comics*, 235.

12. Ibid., 249–50.

13. The reputation of *Understanding Comics* still eclipses that of McCloud's later two books, *Reinventing Comics* and *Making Comics*, both of which in many ways surpass their predecessor. *Understanding Comics* received three Harvey Awards in 1994: Best Writer, Best Graphic Album/Original Material, and Best Biographical, Historical or Journalistic Presentation.

14. Sabin is skeptical of such distant historical origins for comics: "this kind of historical extrapolation is dubious in its logic," he argues, "and often used to 'justify' comics by association with more culturally-respected forms" (*Adult Comics*, 13). McCloud's ambitious historical claims were part of his effort to transform the common perception of comics as a disposable and juvenile medium.

15. For a more theoretical discussion of comics as a visual system, see Groensteen's *System of Comics*, *Comics and Narration*, and "Few Words." Hatfield has outlined a set of visual tensions in comics that provides a useful frame for formal analysis in his *Alternative Comics*, 32–67.

16. For critiques of *Understanding Comics*, see Horrocks, "Inventing Comics"; Delany, "Politics"; Miller, review of *Teaching*, 225–28; and Witek, review of *Understanding*.

17. Page numbers will be provided parenthetically for subsequent references to Inge's *Comics as Culture*.

18. Harvey, *Art of the Comic Book*, 262. For an early discussion between McCloud and Harvey, see McCloud, "Round and Round."

19. See "Interview with Roger Sabin" by Ernesto Priego, *The Comics Grid* (blog), December 5, 2011, http://blog.comicsgrid.com/2011/12/roger-sabin-interview/.

20. Witek, "Comics Criticism," 11–12.

21. Nelson, *Secret Life*, 79. Despite its errors, the book won the tenth annual Aldo and Jeanne Scaglione Prize for Comparative Literary Studies, sponsored by the Modern Language Association of America.

22. Ibid.

23. See (in chronological order) Baetens, *Graphic Novel*; Varnum and Gibbons, *Language*; Talon, *Panel Discussions*; Gravett, *Manga* and *Graphic Novels*; Brunetti, *Anthology*; Hignite, *In the Studio*; Carter, *Building Literacy*; Wolk, *Reading Comics*; Versaci, *This Book*; Heer and Worcester, *Comics Studies Reader*; Duncan and Smith, *Power of Comics*; Tabachnick, *Teaching*; Weiner, *Graphic Novels*; Petersen, *Comics, Manga*; Gravett, *1001 Comics*; Irving and Kushner, *Leaping*; and Smith and Duncan, *Critical Approaches*.

24. See (in chronological order) Brown, *Black Superheroes*; Fingeroth, *Disguised*; Baskind and Omer-Sherman, *Jewish Graphic Novel*; Aldama, *Your Brain*; Ahrens and Meteling, *Comics*; Aldama, *Multicultural Comics*; Chute, *Graphic Women*; Prough, *Straight*; and Nama, *Super Black*.

25. Beaty, "In Focus," 108.

26. Catherine Labio has argued that the widespread adoption of "graphic novel" as a catchall for comics in general "reflects a sad narrowing of the field to a very small and unrepresentative canon" ("What's in a Name?," 124). Likewise, Ann Miller has warned that the habitual citation of a few creators (such as Chris Ware, Joe Sacco, and Art Spiegelman) in the MLA's *Teaching the Graphic Novel* "has a certain canon-forming effect" (review of *Teaching*, 223). For one manifestation of the canonical impulse outside of academia, see Spurgeon, "Top 100."

27. See, for example, the exchange between Ben Saunders and Hillary Chute in *PMLA* ("Forum"). Writing in response to Chute's "Comics as Literature?"

from the previous year, Saunders warns against unexamined "aesthetic hierarchies" that shun "genre work in general and superhero stories in particular" (Saunders and Chute, "Forum," 292–95). Chute's response offers a chilly dismissal of Saunders's concerns, and Saunders develops his arguments further in his *Do the Gods*, 144–51. Such disagreements over the relative status of different genres and creators reflect the felt need to qualify comics as "literature" through negative classification.

28. Campbell, "What Is a Graphic Novel?," 13.

29. Labio, "What's in a Name?," 126.

30. Hillary Chute has sensibly suggested that "it is not so important to *define* comics, to construct an excluding box around the medium (this is comics and this is not comics) as to write well about what we consider comics can do, and what work they are accomplishing through various properties peculiar to the form" ("Decoding Comics," 1020).

31. Waugh, *Comics*; McCloud, *Understanding*. See also Witek, "Comics Criticism," 8–10 (on Waugh), and Meskin, "Defining Comics?" (on McCloud).

32. McCloud, *Understanding*, 4–9.

33. Ibid., 5.

34. Horrocks, "Inventing Comics," 31.

35. Aaron Meskin has suggested that "the real function of constructing a closed and ahistorical artistic category that most comics belong to is to establish an ersatz history for comics—one that might legitimate their place in the world of art" ("Defining Comics?," 374).

36. Horrocks, "Inventing Comics," 34. McCloud's emphasis on comics as a visual medium, for example, "implies that pictures should dominate words in comics; narrative should be pictorial, not textual" (ibid.). Horrocks offers examples of prominent amounts of text in comics such as Foster, *Prince*

Valiant, and Sim, *Cerberus*. More recent comics that feature copious text include Bechdel, *Are You My Mother?*, and Hickman, *Nightly News*.

37. Chute, "Comics as Literature?," 452.
38. "Throughout this essay, I treat comics as a medium—not as a lowbrow genre, which is how it is usually understood" (ibid.).
39. For critiques of this trend, see Meskin, "Comics as Literature?," and Miodrag, "Narrative, Language."
40. Versaci, *This Book*, 12.
41. K. Williams, review of *This Book*, 129.
42. See Meskin, "Comics as Literature?," 239.
43. Chute, "Comics as Literature?," 452.
44. Jefferson, *Writings*, 104–5.
45. Tabachnick, "Comic-Book World," 25, 27.
46. Meskin, "Comics as Literature?," 222.
47. Several scholars like Charles Hatfield and Marc Singer are also active bloggers, while other prominent writers such as Paul Gravett maintain a presence online. See Hatfield and Fischer, *Thought Balloonists* (blog), http://seehatfield.typepad.com/; Singer, *I Am NOT the Beastmaster* (blog), http://notthebeastmaster.typepad.com/weblog/; and Gravett's website, http://www.paulgravett.com/ (all accessed September 22, 2013).
48. Smith, "Surveying," 140.
49. Institute, "Welcome."
50. Sequart Research and Literacy Organization, "Books," *Sequart Research and Literacy Organization: Advancing Comics as Art*, http://sequart.org/books/ (accessed September 21, 2013).
51. See Carrier, *Aesthetics*, 62.
52. Comics studies has been always been responsive to such analysis, and recent work shows resurgent interest in multiple contexts and communities. Smith and Duncan, *Critical Approaches*, contains essay clusters on "Production," "Context," and "Reception," for example, while the *Journal of Graphic Novels and Comics* recently devoted an issue to various readerships in comics (Weiner and Gibson, "Audiences").
53. Witek, "Comics Criticism," 15.

Chapter 2

1. Goldwater, Bloom, and Montana, "America's Newest"; DeCarlo, *Archie's Girls*; Buell, *Little Lulu*; Siegel, Shuster, et al., *Superman*; Kane, Finger, et al., *Batman*.
2. Crumb, "Mr. Natural."
3. Trudeau, *Doonesbury*; Bechdel, *Dykes*; Mack, *Stan Mack's*; Feiffer, *Sick Sick Sick*.
4. Larson, *The Far Side*; Johnston, *For Better*.
5. Spiegelman, *Maus*.
6. Tomorrow, "Immortality," 88; Bolling, *Thrilling Tom*, 140.
7. Tomorrow, "Immortality," 88.
8. Squier, *Liminal Lives*, 201–3; 268–70. Page numbers will be provided parenthetically in subsequent references to this text.
9. Ian Williams, Graphic Medicine website, http://www.graphicmedicine.org/ian-williams/ (accessed September 22, 2013).
10. In retrospect, this moment of convergence fascinates me. Comics were marginal to my intellectual agenda in 2006, while at that point Michael was already teaching comics to his medical students (though I wouldn't learn that until years later). And although Kimberly would move to Penn State Hershey in the future, she was not a colleague at that point. The mutual interest in medical humanities that brought my co-authors and I together in 2002 would be reshaped, by 2011, into our collaborative work in graphic medicine.
11. Columbia University Medical Center, Program in Narrative Medicine, College of Physicians and Surgeons, "Mission," *Program in Narrative Medicine*, http://

www.narrativemedicine.org (accessed September 21, 2013). Portions of this essay appeared in Squier, "Case Narrative." For a succinct précis of Montgomery's distinctive contribution to the intellectual discipline of the medical humanities, see Chambers, "Misreading Montgomery."

12. Charon and Montello, *Stories Matter*, ix.

13. Ostherr, "Narrative Medicine," 120.

14. Ostherr, "Narrative Medicine"; Ostherr, *Medical Visions*; Davis and Morris, "Biocultures Manifesto."

15. Halas and Manvell, *Technique*, 134.

16. Charon and Montello, *Stories Matter*, 59. Page numbers will be provided parenthetically in subsequent references to this text.

17. Page numbers will be provided parenthetically for subsequent references to *Mom's Cancer*.

18. My thanks to Andrea Charise and Teresa Mangum for including me in this Working Symposium, and to the other participants, Therese (Tess) Jones, Paul Crawford, Maura Spiegel, Anna Willieme, and Erin Gentry Lamb, for the fascinating discussions. My notes on this discussion are my own and are not necessarily indicative of the formal symposium proceedings to come. See the Obermann Center for Advanced Studies web page describing the symposium, http://obermann.uiowa.edu /news/health-humanities-building-future-research-and-teaching (accessed April 15, 2014).

19. Siebers, "Disability and the Theory." That this is not the only aim of scholarship in DS should perhaps go without saying, but it is still a point worth making. Giving testimony, engaging in imaginative play, challenging normate understandings, catalyzing community, and providing personal and historical documentation are also important aspects of scholarship in DS.

20. Eisner, *Expressive Anatomy*. Eisner initially used this term in the first volume of his series, *Comics and Sequential Art*, which was reissued by Norton in 2008.

21. Eisner, *Comics and Sequential Art*, 100.

22. Leka, *I Am Not These Feet*. This text is not paginated.

23. Satrapi, *Embroideries*. This text is not paginated.

24. See Squier, "Comics in the Health Humanities."

25. Saiya Miller and Liza Bley, *Not Your Mother's Meatloaf* (blog), http://sexed comicproject.blogspot.com (last modified September 15, 2010).

26. Saiya Miller and Liza Bley, eds., *Not Your Mother's Meatloaf* website, http:// notyourmothersmeatloafbook.com (accessed March 24, 2014).

27. Ibid.

28. Saiya Miller, personal interview with author [Susan M. Squier], May 2011.

29. Boston Women's Health Book Collective, *Our Bodies*.

30. American Psychiatric Association, *Diagnostic and Statistical*.

31. Page numbers will be provided parenthetically for subsequent references to *Monsters*.

32. McCay, *Little Nemo*; Sendak, *In the Night*.

33. My thanks to Matt Weber for this observation, from his illuminating reading of Dahl's *Monsters*.

34. Morrison and Quitely, *We3*; Tezuka, *Ode to Kirihito*; Alanguilan, *Elmer*.

35. Barbara Natterson-Horowitz and Kathryn Bowers point out that the separation of animal and human illnesses and treatment is a relatively recent phenomenon, which they date to the late 1800s: "A century or two ago, in some rural communities, animals and humans were cared for by the same practitioner. And physicians and veterinarians both claim the same 19th-century doctor, William Osler, as a father of their fields."

See Natterson-Horowitz and Bowers, "Our Animal Natures."

36. While much ink has been spilled on this topic, here is a good place to start: Cathy Davidson, "The Crisis in the Humanities and STEM—and Why We Must Recreate Higher Education," *DMLCentral: Digital Media + Learning: The Power of Participation* (blog), November 25, 2013, http://dmlcentral .net/blog/cathy-davidson/crisis-hu manities-and-stem-–-and-why-we- must-recreate-higher-education.

37. Brunetti's inductive method of learning to draw and his essayistic, professorial tone are initially engaging, but by the end of the semester his approach to comics can feel limited by its mod- ernist, high-art commitments. (My modernist literary theory students felt somewhat differently, however.) Abel and Madden's textbook is welcoming, very nuts and bolts, and structured like a fifteen-week semester, with reading and drawing assignments for each week. The drawback there is size: the very large-format paperback (8.5 × 14 inches) is clunky to lug to class, if you aren't an art student schlepping a portfolio. But Abel and Madden also have a website and blog where tips are available for anyone wanting to dip into comics creation, and they are remarkably recep- tive to questions and comments from readers. I dream of the day they produce a standard-size version of their textbook for non-art-student readers.

38. See Roselló's website, http://www .jarodrosello.com/ (accessed March 24, 2014). Roselló helped shape the vision of my first comics seminar. He was an MFA candidate when we first collabo- rated; I gave him a directed reading, and in return he guided the studio portion. He is now an assistant professor of cre- ative writing at the University of South Florida, having completed his Ph.D. in Education by submitting an original

graphic novel of two hundred pages and eleven essays on comics and pedagogy.

39. Thanks to Czerwiec for suggesting this formula for a jam comic when I was working with a very bright and cautious group of graduate students: Write a sto- ry underneath the panels, spacing it out so that each panel has part of the story as its caption. The story should start: "People don't know this about me, but I used to. . . ."

40. Abel and Madden have a page on their website that offers suggestions for other types of jam comics, a set of jam comic rules, and a nine-panel grid that you can download. See Abel and Madden, "Activity: The Jam Comic," *Drawing Words and Writing Pictures* website, http://dw-wp.com/2010/07/activi ty-the-jam-comic/ (posted July 7, 2010).

41. Throughout the studio hour, I talk with the students about their experiences of this new process of making comics. I ask them to share the anxieties, pleasures, stumbling blocks, or breakthroughs they experience, and we discuss the implica- tions of those responses for our work as comics studies scholars. In particular, we talk about how our expectations of comics change as we are drawing our own.

42. Adam Perry and his brother Logan Perry presented an early version of their diabetes comic at the 2011 Graphic Medicine conference in Chicago. See Perry and Perry, "Call for Help."

43. Latour, "Why Has Critique," 232. Page numbers will be provided parenthetical- ly for subsequent references to this text.

44. Recently, in a Facebook posting, cartoonist Jessica Abel proposed a workshop in which writers will be able to "use comics panels and grids to assess and revise prose. The idea is to use com- ics' strengths—visual language, pacing, rhythm, concrete action, sequencing, etc.—to process a scene or short story from your prose (or poetry) work." See

Abel, "Revising Prose with Comics Language Workshop/Salon," Facebook post, June 23, 2012, https://www.facebook.com/events/408007822559555/. The very properties essential to comics creation can also invigorate their scholarly writing, as Abel's workshop proposal suggests: the "visual language, pacing, rhythm, concrete action, [and effective] sequencing" of comics are likely to be precisely the lessons graduate students need to learn if they want to write prose that reaches beyond the academy to grab the interest of general readers.

45. Charon, "Honoring Stories."
46. For information about the "funny animals/funny aminals" traditions in comics, see Witek, *Comic Books*.

Chapter 3

1. Throughout this chapter, I tend to avoid using the term "graphic novel" because I associate it with book-length fictional accounts. Instead, I use the term "comics," or "graphic narratives," to refer to the combined use of images and text, sequentially, to tell a story, where the images complement and/or enhance the text (McCloud, *Understanding*, 9). The comics of which I speak are not necessarily funny, fictional, or lengthy, and they address every conceivable topic, serious or otherwise, using a variety of formats. Comics that are memoirs about illness experiences are referred to as "graphic pathographies," a term coined by my colleague Kimberly Myers and me in a *British Medical Journal* article (Green and Myers, "Graphic Medicine," 574). I wish to thank Michael Goldenberg, an undergraduate student at Penn State's Schreyer Honors College, for his assistance with researching the use of comics in higher education.
2. Lee, *Fantastic Four*; Lee and Ditko, *Spider-Man*.

3. Wynn and Elson, *Anatomy Coloring Book*; Goldberg, *Clinical Neuroanatomy*.
4. See Ian Williams's Graphic Medicine website at http://www.graphicmedicine.org/ian-williams/ (accessed September 22, 2013).
5. Macnaughton, "The Humanities," 23–26.
6. Reilly, Ring, and Duke, "Visual Thinking Strategies," 251–52.
7. Kakalios, *Physics*; Gerde and Foster, "X-Men Ethics"; Jacobs, "More than Words."
8. Hosler and Boomer, "Are Comic Books."
9. Rogers and Ford, "Factors."
10. McCloud, *Making Comics*; Gertler and Lieber, *Complete*; Abel and Madden, *Drawing Words*.
11. Gunderman, *Achieving Excellence*, 19, 84.
12. Elliott and Strubberg, "Humanizing."

Chapter 4

1. Spiegelman, *Maus.*
2. Marchetto, *Cancer Vixen.*
3. Crane, "Monster," 6, 38.
4. See Shelley, *Frankenstein.*
5. Page numbers will be provided parenthetically for subsequent references to Marchetto's *Cancer Vixen.*
6. Myers and Mack, "When the Patient Knows."
7. Throughout this experience and the treatments that would follow, I was keenly aware of how privileged I was to have excellent medical professionals who were also personal friends. Although my anxiety was intense, I knew it would have been far worse had I not had insiders who helped me navigate the labyrinthine medical system swiftly and efficiently. I eagerly welcomed this support, yet I also felt somewhat guilty, realizing that most patients would not have such advocacy and encouragement. This realization led me to a commitment to work with women who have been diagnosed with

breast cancer, helping them in whatever ways I can.

Chapter 5

1. Gilman, "AIDS," is the first use of the term "iconography of illness." Throughout the chapter, I use the term "comics," a singular noun used in the plural, to cover both the physical objects (including their extended form, graphic novels) and the attendant philosophy and practice of the medium.
2. Green and Myers, "Graphic," 574. For a fascinating history of this genre, see Sabin, *Comics, Comix.*
3. See, for example, Shelton, *Collected.*
4. Donald, *Viz.*
5. See the Graphic Medicine website, http://www.graphicmedicine.org /ian-williams.
6. Ware, "Introduction," 12.
7. Radley, "Portrayals," 2.
8. Stahl, "Living," 55.
9. W. J. T. Mitchell, *What Do,* xv.
10. Lupton, *Medicine as Culture,* 79.
11. Gilman, *Disease,* 2.
12. Gilman, "AIDS," 88.
13. Walker, *Lexicon,* quoted in Brownlee, "Quimps."
14. Dahl, *Monsters,* 88.
15. Barthes, *Image, Music, Text,* 43.
16. Chute, *Graphic Women,* 193.
17. El Refaie, *Autobiographical Comics,* 8; see also Merleau-Ponty, *Phenomenology,* and Leder, *Absent Body.*
18. Radley, "Portrayals," 2.
19. Ibid.
20. Sontag, *Illness as Metaphor,* 131. For an excellent discussion of stigma, see Goffman, *Stigma.*
21. Small, *Stitches,* 190–91.
22. Small was told that his mother did not love him, as a fact, by his therapist, who knew his mother. He relates the story of the therapist giving him this information in various talks he has given about *Stitches.*
23. The substitution of anthropomorphic animals for humans is a fascinating trope in media such as comics, animation, and children's books.
24. McCloud, *Understanding,* 36.
25. Ibid.
26. See Gilman, *Disease,* 4.
27. Dahl, *Monsters,* 51–52.
28. Gilman, *Disease,* 4.
29. Clinical Effectiveness Group, "2007 National Guideline," 2.
30. Gilman, *Disease,* 4. There has been speculation that this stigmatization of herpes was perpetrated deliberately after acyclovir was invented. Before there was any specific treatment, herpes was just a rash; after treatment was developed, it became a dreaded disease. See Scott, "Courts."
31. Dahl, *Monsters,* 199.
32. The idea of "the other" was formalized by Emmanuel Levinas and later made popular by Edward Said in his well-known book *Orientalism.*
33. Ferrier, *Disrepute.*
34. Davis, "Suffering," 64.
35. Ibid., 76.
36. Ibid., 62–77.
37. A. Mitchell, "Distributed Identity," 258.
38. For a documentary film that provides an excruciating overview of Flanagan's work, see Kirby, *Sick.*

Chapter 6

Student art and comments used with permission.

1. Kelley, *And Then What,* 151.
2. Torrance, *Understanding,* 3.
3. Barry, *What It Is,* 80.
4. Barry, "Doodle Your Way."
5. Leavitt, "Nonfiction."
6. Ebert, "You Can Draw, and Probably Better than I Can," *Roger Ebert.com,* February 25, 2011, http://www.roger ebert.com/rogers-journal/you-can-draw-and-probably-better-than-i-can.
7. Charon, *Narrative Medicine,* 156.

8. Montello, "Narrative Ethics."

9. Abel and Madden, *Drawing Words*, 13.

10. Barry, *What It Is*, 143–53.

11. Nicole Rudick, "Lynda Barry on 'Picture This,'" *The Paris Review Daily* (blog), December 1, 2010, http://www .theparisreview.org/blog/2010/12/01 /lynda-barry-on-picture-this/.

12. Brunetti, *Cartooning*, 5.

13. Quoted in ibid., 66.

14. Milner, *On Not Being*, 142.

15. Czerwiec, "Narrative Constipation,"18.

16. Green and Rieck, "Missed It," 357–61.

17. Michael J. Green, personal correspondence with author [MK Czerwiec], April 26, 2013.

18. Ibid.

19. Kelly, "What Are You Doing," 1476.

20. Ibid.

21. Al-Jawad, personal interview with author [MK Czerwiec], July 19, 2012.

22. Al-Jawad, "Comics Are Research."

23. Al-Jawad, personal interview.

24. Charon, *Narrative Medicine*, 156.

SELECTED BIBLIOGRAPHY

Abel, Jessica, and Matt Madden. *Drawing Words and Writing Pictures: Making Comics; Manga, Graphic Novels, and Beyond.* New York: First Second, 2008.

Ahrens, Jörn, and Arno Meteling. *Comics and the City: Urban Space in Print, Picture, and Sequence.* New York: Continuum, 2010.

Aldama, Frederick Luis, ed. *Multicultural Comics: From Zap to Blue Beetle.* Austin: University of Texas Press, 2010.

———. *Your Brain on Latino Comics: From Gus Arriola to Los Bros Hernandez.* Austin: University of Texas Press, 2009.

Al-Jawad, Muna. "Comics Are Research: Graphic Narratives as a New Way of Seeing Clinical Practice." *Journal of Medical Humanities,* February 2, 2013. doi: 10.1007/s10912-013-9205-0.

Al-Jawad, Muna. *Old Person Whisperer* (blog). HYPERLINK "http://oldperson whisperer.tumblr.com/"http:// oldpersonwhisperer.tumblr.com / (accessed February 3, 2014).

American Psychiatric Association. *Diagnostic and Statistical Manual of Mental Disorders: DSM-5.* 5th ed. Washington, DC: American Psychiatric Association, 2013.

Ault, Donald, ed. *ImageText: Interdisciplinary Comics Studies.* Gainesville: Department of English, University of Florida, 2004–. http://www .english.ufl.edu/imagetext/.

Baetens, Jan, ed. *The Graphic Novel.* Louvain, Belgium: Leuven University Press, 2001.

Barker, Martin. *A Haunt of Fears: The Strange History of the British Horror Comics Campaign.* London: Pluto Press, 1984.

Barry, Lynda. "Doodle Your Way Out of Writer's Block." Interview by Neal Conan. National Public Radio, *Talk of the Nation,* November 11, 2010. http://www.npr .org/2010/11/11/131247663/doodle- your-way-out-of-writer-s-block.

Barthes, Roland. *Image, Music, Text.* Translated by Stephen Heath. 1st pbk. ed. New York: Farrar, Straus and Giroux, 1978.

Baskind, Samantha, and Ranen Omer- Sherman, eds. *The Jewish Graphic Novel: Critical Approaches.* New Brunswick: Rutgers University Press, 2008.

Beaty, Bart. *Fredric Wertham and the Critique of Mass Culture.* Jackson: University Press of Mississippi, 2005.

———, ed. "In Focus: Comics Studies; Fifty Years After Film Studies." Special section, *Cinema Journal* 50, no. 3 (Spring 2011): 106–34.

Boston Women's Health Book Collective. *Our Bodies, Our Selves: A Book by and for Women*. 1st ed. Boston: New England Free Press, 1971.

Boyer, Ernest L. *Scholarship Reconsidered: Priorities of the Professoriate*. Princeton, NJ: The Carnegie Foundation for the Advancement of Teaching, 1990.

Brown, Jeffrey A. *Black Superheroes, Milestone Comics, and Their Fans*. Jackson: University Press of Mississippi, 2001.

Brownlee, John. "Quimps, Plewds, and Grawlixes: The Secret Language of Comic Strips." *Co.Design*. Posted July 15, 2013. http://www.fastcodesign.com/1673017/quimps-plewds-and-grawlixes-the-secret-language-of-comic-strips.

Brunetti, Ivan, ed. *An Anthology of Graphic Fiction, Cartoons, and True Stories*. 2 vols. New Haven: Yale University Press, 2006–8.

———. *Cartooning: Philosophy and Practice*. New Haven: Yale University Press, 2011.

Campbell, Eddie. "What Is a Graphic Novel?" *World Literature Today* 81, no. 2 (March–April 2007): 13.

Carrier, David. *The Aesthetics of Comics*. University Park: The Pennsylvania State University Press, 2000.

Carter, James Bucky, ed. *Building Literacy Connections with Graphic Novels: Page by Page, Panel by Panel*. Urbana, IL: National Council of Teachers of Education, 2007.

Chapman, Robyn. *Drawing Comics Lab: 52 Exercises on Characters, Panels, Storytelling, Publishing, and Professional Practices*. Beverly, MA: Quarry Books, 2012.

Charon, Rita. "Honoring Stories of Illness." Lecture, TEDxAtlanta. Posted November 4, 2011. http://www.youtube.com/watch?feature=player_embedded&v=24kHX2HtU3o.

———. *Narrative Medicine*. Oxford: Oxford University Press, 2006.

Charon, Rita, and Martha Montello, eds. *Stories Matter: The Role of Narrative in Medical Ethics*. New York: Routledge, 2002.

Chute, Hillary L. "Comics as Literature? Reading Graphic Narrative." *PMLA* 123, no. 2 (March 2008): 452–65.

———. "Decoding Comics." *MFS: Modern Fiction Studies* 52, no. 4 (Winter 2006): 1014–27.

———. *Graphic Women: Life Narrative and Contemporary Comics*. New York: Columbia University Press, 2010.

Clinical Effectiveness Group (British Association for Sexual Health and HIV). "2007 National Guideline for the Management of Genital Herpes." *British Association for Sexual Health and HIV*. http://www.bashh.org/documents/115/115.pdf (accessed May 5, 2013).

Comics Grid: The Journal of Comics Scholarship. London: Ubiquity Press, 2013–. http://www.comicsgrid.com/.

Cooke, Jon B., ed. *Comic Book Artist*. Raleigh, NC: TwoMorrows Publishing, 1998–2002; Marietta, GA: Top Shelf Productions, 2003–5.

Crane, Stephen. "The Monster." In *"The Monster" and Other Stories*, 3–106. New York: Harper and Brothers, 1899.

Czerwiec, MK. "Narrative Constipation." *Atrium: The Report of the Northwestern Medical Humanities and Bioethics Program* 7 (2009): 16–18. http://bioethics.northwestern.edu/atrium/pdf/atrium-issue7.pdf/.

Davis, Joseph E. "Suffering, Pharmaceutical Advertising, and the Face of Mental Illness." *The Hedgehog Review* 8, no. 3 (Fall 2006): 62–77.

Davis, Lennard J., and David B. Morris. "Biocultures Manifesto." *New Literary History* 38, no. 3 (Summer 2007): 411–18.

Delany, Samuel R. "The Politics of Paraliterary Criticism." In *Shorter Views: Queer Thoughts and the Politics of the Paraliterary*, 218–70. Hanover: University Press of New England, 1999.

Duncan, Randy, and Matthew J. Smith. *The Power of Comics: History, Form, and Culture*. New York: Continuum, 2009.

Eisner, Will. *Comics and Sequential Art*. Tamarack, FL: Poorhouse Press, 1985.

———. *Expressive Anatomy for Comics and Narrative: Principles and Practices from the Legendary Cartoonist*. New York: W. W. Norton, 2008.

Elliott, Tim, and Brandon Strubberg. "Humanizing Medicine Through Graphic Storytelling: A Rhetorical Analysis of Student-Created Graphic Narratives." Paper presented at the international conference Comics and Medicine: Navigating the Margins, Toronto, July 22–23, 2012.

El Refaie, Elisabeth. *Autobiographical Comics: Life Writing in Pictures*. Jackson: University Press of Mississippi, 2012.

European Comic Art. New York: Berghahn Books, 2008–.

Ewing, William A. *The Body: Photographs of the Human Form*. San Francisco: Chronicle Books, 1994.

Feiffer, Jules. *The Great Comic Book Heroes*. New York: Dial Press, 1965.

Fingeroth, Danny. *Disguised as Clark Kent: Jews, Comics, and the Creation of the Superhero*. New York: Continuum, 2007.

Gabilliet, Jean-Paul. *Of Comics and Men: A Cultural History of American Comic Books*. Translated by Bart Beaty and Nick Nguyen. Jackson: University Press of Mississippi, 2010. Originally published as *Des comics et des hommes: Histoire culturelle des comic books aux États-Unis*. Paris: Editions du Temps, 2005.

Gerde, Virginia W., and R. Spencer Foster. "X-Men Ethics: Using Comic Books to Teach Business Ethics." *Journal of Business Ethics* 77, no. 3 (February 2008): 245–58.

Gertler, Nat, and Steve Lieber. *The Complete Idiot's Guide to Creating a Graphic Novel*. New York: Alpha Books, 2004.

Gilman, Sander L. "AIDS and Syphilis: The Iconography of Disease." In "AIDS: Cultural Analysis/Cultural Activism," edited by Douglas Crimp. Special issue, *October* 43 (Winter 1987): 87–107.

———. *Disease and Representation: Images of Illness from Madness to AIDS*. Ithaca: Cornell University Press, 1988.

Goffman, Erving. *Stigma: Notes on the Management of Spoiled Identity*. New York: Touchstone, 1986.

Goldberg, Stephen. *Clinical Neuroanatomy Made Ridiculously Simple*. Miami: MedMaster, 1979.

Gravett, Paul. *Graphic Novels: Everything You Need to Know*. New York: Harper Design, 2005.

———. *Manga: Sixty Years of Japanese Comics*. London: Laurence King Publishing, 2004.

———, ed. *1001 Comics You Must Read Before You Die: The Ultimate Guide to Comic Books, Graphic Novels, and Manga*. New York: Universe, 2011.

Green, Michael J., and Kimberly Myers. "Graphic Medicine: Use of Comics in Medical Education and Patient Care." *British Medical Journal* 340 (March 13, 2010): 474–77.

Groensteen, Thierry. *Comics and Narration*. Translated by Ann Miller. Jackson: University Press of Mississippi, 2013. Originally published as *Bande dessinée et narration*, vol. 2 of *Système de la bande dessinée*. Paris: Presses Universitaires de France, 2011.

———. "A Few Words About *The System of Comics* and More. . . ." *European Comic Art* 1, no. 1 (June 6, 2008): 87–95.

———. *The System of Comics*. Translated by Bart Beaty and Nick Nguyen. Jackson: University Press of Mississippi, 2007. Originally published as *Système de la bande dessinée*. Paris: Presses Universitaires de France, 1999.

Groth, Gary, ed. *The Comics Journal*. Seattle, WA: Fantagraphics Books, 1977–. [Formerly *The New Nostalgia Journal*.]

Gunderman, Richard B. *Achieving Excellence in Medical Education*. London: Springer, 2011.

Hajdu, David. *The Ten-Cent Plague: The Great Comic-Book Scare and How It Changed America*. New York: Farrar, Straus and Giroux, 2008.

Halas, John, and Roger Manvell. *The Technique of Film Animation*. 2nd ed. New York: Hastings House, 1968.

Harvey, Robert C. *The Art of the Comic Book: An Aesthetic History*. Jackson: University Press of Mississippi, 1996.

———. *The Art of the Funnies: An Aesthetic History*. Jackson: University Press of Mississippi, 1994.

Hatfield, Charles. *Alternative Comics: An Emerging Literature*. Jackson: University Press of Mississippi, 2005.

———. "Defining Comics in the Classroom; or, The Pros and Cons of Unfixability." In *Teaching the Graphic Novel*, edited by Stephen E. Tabachnick, 19–27. New York: The Modern Language Association of America, 2009.

Heer, Jeet, and Kent Worcester, eds. *Arguing Comics: Literary Masters on a Popular Medium*. Jackson: University Press of Mississippi, 2004.

———. *A Comics Studies Reader*. Jackson: University Press of Mississippi, 2009.

Hignite, Todd, ed. *Comic Art*. Oakland, CA: Buenaventura Press, 2002–7.

———. *In the Studio: Visits with Contemporary Cartoonists*. New Haven: Yale University Press, 2006.

Horrocks, Dylan. "Inventing Comics: Scott McCloud Defines the Form in *Understanding Comics*." *Comics Journal* 234 (June 2001): 29–39.

Hosler, Jay, and K. B. Boomer. "Are Comic Books an Effective Way to Engage Nonmajors in Learning and Appreciating Science?" *CBE: Life Sciences Education* 10, no. 3 (Fall 2011): 309–17.

Image and Narrative. Flanders, Belgium: Open Humanities Press, 2000–. http://www.imageandnarrative.be/index.php/imagenarrative/index.

Inge, M. Thomas. *Comics as Culture*. Jackson: University Press of Mississippi, 1990.

Institute for Comics Studies. "Welcome to the Institute for Comics Studies." *Institute for Comics Studies: Promoting the Study, Understanding, Recognition, and Cultural Legitimacy of Comics*. http://www.instituteforcomicsstudies.org/ (accessed June 4, 2013).

Irving, Christopher, and Seth Kushner. *Leaping Tall Buildings: The Origins of American Comics*. Brooklyn, NY: PowerHouse Books, 2012.

Jacobs, Dale. "More than Words: Comics as a Means of Teaching Multiple Literacies." *The English Journal* 96, no. 3 (January 2007): 19–25.

Jefferson, Thomas. Thomas Jefferson to Nathaniel Burwell, March 14, 1818. In *The Writings of Thomas Jefferson*, vol. 10, *1816–1826*, edited by Paul Leicester Ford, 104–5. New York: G. P. Putnam's Sons, 1899.

Jones, Gerard. *Men of Tomorrow: Geeks, Gangsters, and the Birth of the Comic Book*. New York: Basic Books, 2004.

Journal of Graphic Novels and Comics. London: Taylor and Francis, 2010–.

Kakalios, James. *The Physics of Superheroes*. New York: Gotham Books, 2005.

Katz, Lisa. "Reconstruction." In *Breast Art. The Drunken Boat* 3, no. 1 (Spring 2002). http://www.thedrunkenboat.com /katz.html.

Kelley, Victor. *. . . And Then What Happened?* Bloomington, IN: AuthorHouse, 2013.

Kelly, Niamh. "What Are You Doing Creatively These Days?" *Academic Medicine* 87, no. 11 (November 2012): 1476.

Kirby, Dick, dir. *Sick: The Life and Death of Bob Flanagan, Supermasochist*. Santa Monica, CA: Lion's Gate Entertainment, 2007.

Kunzle, David. *The Early Comic Strip: Narrative Strips and Picture Stories in the European Broadsheet from c. 1450 to 1825*. Berkeley: University of California Press, 1973.

———. *The History of the Comic Strip: The Nineteenth Century*. Berkeley: University of California Press, 1990.

Labio, Catherine. "What's in a Name? The Academic Study of Comics and the 'Graphic Novel.'" *Cinema Journal* 50, no. 3 (Spring 2011): 123–26.

Latour, Bruno. "Why Has Critique Run Out of Steam? From Matters of Fact to Matters of Concern." *Critical Inquiry* 30, no. 2 (Winter 2004): 225–48.

Leavitt, Sarah. "Nonfiction Writer Jam." Lecture, LitFest: Edmonton's Nonfiction Festival, Edmonton, Canada, October 23, 2010. http://www.youtube.com /watch?v=L3llMixmoKk.

Leder, Drew. *The Absent Body*. Chicago: University of Chicago Press, 1990.

Lent, John A., ed. *International Journal of Comic Art*. Drexel Hill, PA: John Lent, 1999–.

Lupton, Deborah. Medicine as Culture: Illness, Disease, and the Body in Western Societies. 2nd ed. London: Sage, 2003.

Macnaughton, Jane. "The Humanities in Medical Education: Context, Outcomes, and Structures." *Medical Humanities* 26, no. 1 (June 2000): 23–30.

Matuschka [Joanne Matuska]. *Beauty Out of Damage*, 1993. Photograph. Multiple galleries. http://www.beautyoutof damage.com/ (accessed September 22, 2013).

McCloud, Scott. *Making Comics: Storytelling Secrets of Comics, Manga, and Graphic Novels*. New York: HarperCollins, 2006.

———. *Reinventing Comics*. New York: Perennial, 2000.

———. "Round and Round with Scott McCloud." Interview by R. C. Harvey. *The Comics Journal* 179 (August 1995): 52–81.

———. *Understanding Comics: The Invisible Art*. New York: HarperPerennial, 1993.

Merleau-Ponty, Maurice. *Phenomenology of Perception*. Translated by Colin Smith. New York: Humanities Press, 1962.

Meskin, Aaron. "Comics as Literature?" *British Journal of Aesthetics* 49, no. 3 (July 2009): 219–39.

———. "Defining Comics?" *Journal of Aesthetics and Art Criticism* 65, no. 4 (Autumn 2007): 369–79.

Miller, Ann. Review of *Teaching the Graphic Novel*, by Stephen E. Tabachnick. *European Comic Art* 3, no. 2 (Autumn 2010): 223–28.

Milner, Marion. *On Not Being Able to Paint*. New York: Routledge, 2011.

Miodrag, Hannah. "Narrative, Language, and Comics-as-Literature." *Studies in Comics* 2, no. 2 (January 2012): 263–79.

Mitchell, Adrielle Anna. "Distributed Identity: Networking Image Fragments in Graphic Memoirs." *Studies in Comics* 1, no. 2 (November 2010): 257–79.

Mitchell, W. J. T. *What Do Pictures Want? The Lives and Loves of Images.* Chicago: University of Chicago Press, 2005.

Montello, Martha. "Narrative Ethics: Making It Practical." Paper presented at the annual meeting of the American Association of Bioethics and Humanities, Washington, DC, October 18–21, 2012.

Myers, Kimberly. *Illness in the Academy: A Collection of Pathographies by Academics.* West Lafayette: Purdue University Press, 2007.

Myers, Kimberly, and Julie Mack. "When the Patient Knows What the Doctor Does Not (Yet) Know." *Atrium: The Report of the Northwestern Medical Humanities and Bioethics Program* 11 (Winter 2013): 19–23.

Nama, Adilifu. *Super Black: American Pop Culture and Black Superheroes.* Austin: University of Texas Press, 2011.

Natterson-Horowitz, Barbara, and Kathryn Bowers. "Our Animal Natures." *New York Times,* Sunday Review, June 10, 2012, SR1. http://www.nytimes.com/2012/06/10/opinion/sunday/our-animal-natures.html?pagewanted=all.

Nelson, Victoria. *The Secret Life of Puppets.* Cambridge, MA: Harvard University Press, 2001.

Nyberg, Amy Kiste. *Seal of Approval: The History of the Comics Code.* Jackson: University Press of Mississippi, 1998.

Ostherr, Kirsten. *Medical Visions: Producing the Patient Through Film, Television, and Imaging Technologies.* New York: Oxford, 2013.

———. "Narrative Medicine, Biocultures, and the Visualization of Health and Disease." In *A Companion to American Literary Studies,* edited by Caroline F. Levander and Robert S. Levine, 108–24. Malden, MA: Wiley-Blackwell, 2001.

Perry, Adam, and Logan Perry. "A Call for Help: Diabetes and Comics." Paper presented at the international conference Comics and Medicine: The Sequential Art of Illness, Chicago, July 9–11, 2011.

Petersen, Robert S. *Comics, Manga, and Graphic Novels: A History of Graphic Narratives.* Santa Barbara, CA: Praeger, 2011.

Prough, Jennifer S. *Straight from the Heart: Gender, Intimacy, and the Cultural Production of Shojo Manga.* Honolulu: University of Hawai'i Press, 2011.

Radley, Alan. "Portrayals of Suffering: On Looking Away, Looking At, and the Comprehension of Illness Experience." *Body and Society* 8, no. 1 (2002): 1–23.

Reilly, Jo Marie, Jeffrey Ring, and Linda Duke. "Visual Thinking Strategies: A New Role for Art in Medical Education." *Family Medicine* 37, no. 4 (April 2005): 250–52.

Rogers, William D., and Robert Ford. "Factors that Affect Student Attitude Toward Biology." *Bioscene* 23, no. 2 (August 1997): 3–5.

Rubenstein, Anne. *Bad Language, Naked Ladies, and Other Threats to the Nation: A Political History of Comic Books in Mexico.* Durham: Duke University Press, 1998.

Sabin, Roger. *Adult Comics: An Introduction.* New York: Routledge, 1993.

———. *Comics, Comix, and Graphic Novels: A History of Comic Art.* London: Phaidon, 1996.

Said, Edward. *Orientalism.* London: Routledge and Kegan Paul, 1978.

Saunders, Ben. *Do the Gods Wear Capes? Spirituality, Fantasy, and Superheroes.* London: Continuum, 2011.

selected
bibliography

187

Saunders, Ben, and Hillary Chute. "Forum: Divisions in Comics Scholarship." *PMLA* 124, no. 1 (January 2009): 292–95.

Scott, Nigel. "The Courts Should Keep Out of Our Sex Lives." *spiked*, September 1, 2011. http://www.spiked-online.com/newsite/article/11041#.

Shelley, Mary Wollstonecraft. *Frankenstein; or, The Modern Prometheus.* Edited by J. Paul Hunter. 2nd ed. Norton Critical Editions. New York: W. W. Norton, 2011.

Siebers, Tobin. "Disability and the Theory of Complex Embodiment—For Identity Politics in a New Register." In *The Disability Studies Reader*, edited by Lennard J. Davis, 4th ed., 278–97. New York: Routledge, 2013.

Smith, Greg M. "It Ain't Easy Studying Comics." *Cinema Journal* 50, no. 3 (Spring 2011): 110–12.

———. "Surveying the World of Contemporary Comics Scholarship: A Conversation." *Cinema Journal* 50, no. 3 (Spring 2011): 135–47.

Smith, Matthew J., and Randy Duncan, eds. *Critical Approaches to Comics: Theories and Methods.* New York: Routledge, 2012.

Sontag, Susan. *"Illness as Metaphor" and "AIDS and Its Metaphors."* New York: Doubleday, 1990.

Spiegelman, Art. "An Evening with Art Spiegelman at the Central Library." Interview by Nancy Pearl. *The Seattle Public Library Podcast.* Podcast audio. October 8, 2011. http://seattle.bibliocommons.com/item/show/2906423030_an_evening_with_art_spiegelman_at_the_central_library.

Spurgeon, Tom. "The Top 100 (English-Language) Comics of the Century." *The Comics Journal* 210 (February 1999): 34–113.

Squier, Susan Merrill. *Babies in Bottles: Twentieth-Century Visions of Reproductive Technology.* New Brunswick: Rutgers University Press, 1994.

———. "Case Narrative and Objectivity, Chickens and Comics: My Story About Kathryn Montgomery." *Atrium: The Report of the Northwestern Medical Humanities and Bioethics Program* 11 (Winter 2013): 32–34.

———. "Comics in the Health Humanities: A New Approach to Sex and Gender Education." In *Health Humanities Reader*, edited by Therese Jones, Delese Wear, Lester D. Friedman, and Kathleen Pachucki. New Brunswick: Rutgers University Press, 2014.

———. *Liminal Lives: Imagining the Human at the Frontiers of Biomedicine.* Durham: Duke University Press, 2004.

Stahl, Devan. "Living into the Imagined Body: How the Diagnostic Image Confronts the Lived Body." *Medical Humanities* 39, no. 1 (March 2013): 53–58.

Starr, Ann, and Susan Merrill Squier. "Speaking Women's Bodies: A Conversation." *Literature and Medicine* 17, no. 2 (Fall 1998): 231–54.

Studies in Comics. Bristol, England: Intellect, 2010–.

Tabachnick, Stephen E. "A Comic-Book World." *World Literature Today* 81, no. 2 (March–April 2007): 24–28.

———, ed. *Teaching the Graphic Novel.* New York: The Modern Language Association of America, 2009.

Talon, Durwin S. *Panel Discussions: Design in Sequential Art Storytelling.* Raleigh, NC: TwoMorrows Publishing, 2007.

Torrance, E. Paul. *Understanding the Fourth Grade Slump in Creative Thinking: Final Report.* Minneapolis: University of Minnesota, 1967.

Van Lente, Fred, and Ryan Dunlavey. *The Comic Book History of Comics: The Inspiring, Infuriating, and Utterly*

Insane Story of the American Comic Book Industry. San Diego, CA: IDW Publishing, 2012.

Varnum, Robin, and Christina T. Gibbons, eds. *The Language of Comics: Word and Image.* Jackson: University Press of Mississippi, 2001.

Versaci, Rocco. *This Book Contains Graphic Language: Comics as Literature.* New York: Continuum, 2007.

Walker, Mort. *The Lexicon of Comicana.* Bloomington, IN: iUniverse, 2000.

Ware, Chris. "Introduction." In *McSweeney's Quarterly Concern: An Assorted Sampler of North American Comic Drawings, Strips, and Illustrated Stories,* no. 13, edited by Chris Ware, 8–12. San Francisco: McSweeney's Quarterly, 2004.

Waugh, Coulton. *The Comics.* New York: Macmillan, 1947.

Weiner, Robert G., ed. *Graphic Novels in Libraries and Archives: Essays on Readers, Research, History, and Cataloging.* Jefferson, NC: McFarland, 2010.

Weiner, Robert G., and Mel Gibson, eds. "Audiences and Readership." Special issue, *Journal of Graphic Novels and Comics* 2, no. 2 (December 2011).

Williams, Kristian. Review of *This Book Contains Graphic Language: Comics as Literature,* by Rocco Versaci. *The Comics Journal* 294 (December 2008): 129–31.

Witek, Joseph. *Comic Books as History: The Narrative Art of Jack Jackson, Art Spiegelman, and Harvey Pekar.* Jackson: University Press of Mississippi, 1989.

———. "Comics Criticism in the United States: A Brief Historical Survey." *International Journal of Comic Art* 1, no. 1 (Spring/Summer 1999): 4–16.

———. Review of *Understanding Comics,* by Scott McCloud. *Inks: Cartoon and Comic Art Studies* 1, no. 1 (February 1994): 42–47.

Wolk, Douglas. *Reading Comics: How Graphic Novels Work and What They Mean.* Boston: Da Capo Press, 2007.

Word and Image: A Journal of Verbal/Visual Enquiry. London: Taylor and Francis, 1985–.

Wright, Bradford W. *Comic Book Nation: The Transformation of Youth Culture in America.* Baltimore: Johns Hopkins University Press, 2001.

Zorbaugh, Harvey, ed. "The Comics as an Educational Medium." Special issue, *Journal of Educational Sociology* 18, no. 4 (Winter 1944).

COMICS BIBLIOGRAPHY

Alanguilan, Gerry. *Elmer: A Comic Book*. San Jose, CA: Slave Labor Graphics, 2010.

Al-Jawad, Muna. *Old Person Whisperer* (blog). http://oldpersonwhisperer.tumblr.com/ (accessed February 3, 2014).

Amazing Stories. New York: Experimenter Publishing [later Teck Publications, Universal Publishing Company, TSR Inc., Wizards of the Coast, Paizo Publishing], 1926–2005.

B., David. *Epileptic*. New York: Pantheon Books, 2006.

Barrier, Michael, and Martin Williams, eds. *A Smithsonian Book of Comic-Book Comics*. Washington, DC: Smithsonian Institution Press, 1981.

Barry, Lynda. *Ernie Pook's Comeek*. Syndicated, 1977–2008.

———. *What It Is*. Montreal: Drawn & Quarterly, 2008.

The Beano. London: D. C. Thomson, 1938–.

Bechdel, Alison. *Are You My Mother?* Boston: Houghton Mifflin Harcourt, 2012.

———. *Dykes to Watch Out For*. Syndicated, 1987–2008.

———. *Fun Home*. Boston: Houghton Mifflin, 2006.

Binder, Otto, Al Plastino, et al. *Legion of Super-Heroes. Adventure Comics*, vol. 1. New York: DC Comics, 1958–83.

Blackbeard, Bill, and Martin Williams, eds. *The Smithsonian Collection of Newspaper Comics*. Washington, DC: Smithsonian Institution Press, 1977.

Bolling, Ruben. *Thrilling Tom the Dancing Bug Stories: A Collection of the Weekly Comic Strip "Tom the Dancing Bug."* Kansas City, MO: Andrews McMeel, 2004.

Brodsky, Sol. *Cracked*. New York: Major Publications, 1958–2007.

Buell, Marjorie Henderson. *Little Lulu. The Saturday Evening Post,* 1935–44.

Burns, Charles. *Black Hole*. Northampton, MA: Kitchen Sink Press, 1995–2005.

Chadwick, Paul. *Concrete*. Vol. 1. Milwaukie, OR: Dark Horse, 1987.

Claremont, Chris, and John Byrne. *The Uncanny X-Men*. Nos. 108–9, 111–43. New York: Marvel Comics, 1977–81.

Corben, Richard, and Robert E. Howard. *Bloodstar*. Leawood, KS: Morning Star Press, 1976.

Crumb, Robert. "Mr. Natural: The Zen Master." *Yarrowstalks* 1 (June 1967): 14.

Cunningham, Darryl. *Psychiatric Tales: Eleven Graphic Stories About Mental Illness*. London: Blank Slate Books, 2010.

Dahl, Ken. *Monsters*. New York: Secret Acres, 2009.

The Dandy Comic. London: D. C. Thomson, 1937–2012.

DeCarlo, Dan. *Archie's Girls Betty and Veronica* [later *Betty and Veronica*]. Mamaroneck, NY: Archie Comics, 1950–.

DeMatteis, J. M., Jon Muth, Kent Williams, and George Pratt. *Moonshadow*. New York: Epic Comics, 1985–87.

Dillon, Glyn. *The Nao of Brown*. London: SelfMadeHero, 2012.

Dirks, Rudolph, et al. *The Katzenjammer Kids*. Syndicated, 1897–.

Donald, Chris, et al. *Viz*. London: Dennis Publishing, 1979–.

Dracula Lives! New York: Curtis Magazines [later Marvel Comics], 1973–75.

Eisner, Will. *A Contract with God and Other Tenement Stories*. New York: Baronet Books, 1978.

Engelberg, Miriam. *Cancer Made Me a Shallower Person: A Memoir in Comics*. New York: Harper, 2006.

Ennis, Garth, and Steve Dillon. *Preacher*. New York: Vertigo [DC Comics], 1995–2000.

Eury, Michael, ed. *Back Issue*. Raleigh, NC: TwoMorrows Publishing, 2003–.

Farmer, Joyce. *Special Exits*. Seattle: Fantagraphics Books, 2010.

Feiffer, Jules. *Sick Sick Sick* [later *Feiffer's Fables; Feiffer*]. *The Village Voice*, 1956–2000.

Ferrier, Thom [Ian Williams]. *Disrepute*. Llanrhaeadr, Wales: Graphic Medicine, 2012.

Fies, Brian. *Mom's Cancer*. New York: Abrams Image, 2006.

Forney, Ellen. *Marbles: Mania, Depression, Michelangelo, and Me; A Graphic Memoir*. New York: Gotham Books, 2012.

Foster, Hal, et al. *Prince Valiant in the Days of King Arthur*. Syndicated, 1937–.

Gaiman, Neil, et al. *The Sandman*. New York: Vertigo [DC Comics], 1989–96.

Gerber, Steve, Frank Brunner, Gene Colan, et al. *Howard the Duck*. New York: Marvel Comics, 1976–79.

Godfrey, Andrew. *The CF Diaries*. Bristol, England: Sicker Than Thou Industries, 2011.

Goldwater, John L., Vic Bloom, and Bob Montana. "America's Newest Boy Friend." *Pep Comics* [later *Archie Comics*] 22 (December 1941).

Green, Justin. *Binky Brown Meets the Holy Virgin Mary*. San Francisco: Last Gasp, 1972.

Green, Michael J., and Ray Rieck. "Missed It." *Annals of Internal Medicine* 158, no. 5 (March 5, 2013): 357–61.

Hernandez, Gilbert, and Jaime Hernandez. *Love and Rockets*. Seattle: Fantagraphics Books, 1982–96, 2001–.

Hickman, Jonathan. *The Nightly News*. Berkeley, CA: Image Comics, 2006–7.

Hosler, Jay. *Optical Allusions*. Columbus, OH: Active Synapse Comics, 2008.

Kane, Bob, Bill Finger, et al. *Batman*. Vol. 1. New York: DC Comics, 1940–2011.

Kochalka, James. *The Cute Manifesto*. Gainesville, FL: Alternative Comics, 2005.

Kurtzman, Harvey. *MAD*. New York: Entertaining Comics [later Kinney Parking Company; DC Comics/Time Warner], 1952–.

Larson, Gary. *The Far Side*. Syndicated, 1980–95.

Leavitt, Sarah. *Tangles: A Story About Alzheimer's, My Mother, and Me*. New York: Skyhorse Publishing, 2012.

Lee, Stan, and Steve Ditko. *Spider-Man. Amazing Fantasy* 15 (August 1962).

Lee, Stan, Bill Everett, et al. *Daredevil*. Vol. 1. New York: Marvel Comics, 1964–98, 2009–11.

Lee, Stan, Jack Kirby, et al. *The Fantastic Four*. Vol. 1. New York: Marvel Comics, 1961–96, 2002–7.

Leka, Kaisa. *I Am Not These Feet*. Helsinki: Absolute Truth Press, 2008.

Linthout, Willy. *Years of the Elephant*. Translated by Michiel Horn. Wisbech, England: Fanfare/Ponent Mon, 2009.

Mack, Stan. *Stan Mack's Real Life Funnies*. *The Village Voice*, 1974–95.

Mackintosh, Ross. *Seeds*. London: Com.x, 2011.

Marchetto, Marisa Acocella. *Cancer Vixen: A True Story*. New York: Alfred A. Knopf, 2006.

McCay, Winsor. *Little Nemo in Slumberland*. *The New York Herald*, 1905–11, 1924–26.

Miller, Frank, and Klaus Janson. *Batman: The Dark Knight Returns*. New York: DC Comics, 1986.

Miller, Frank, and Bill Sienkiewicz. *Elektra: Assassin*. New York: Epic Comics, 1986–87.

Miller, Saiya, and Liza Bley, eds. *Not Your Mother's Meatloaf: A Sex Education Comic Book*. Berkeley, CA: Soft Skull Press, 2013.

Mills, Pat, and John Wagner. *2000AD*. London: IPC Magazines [later Fleetway Publications]; Oxford: Rebellion Developments, 1977–.

Moore, Alan, Dave Gibbons, and John Higgins. *Watchmen*. New York: DC Comics, 1986–87.

Morrison, Grant, and Frank Quitely. *We3*. New York: DC Comics, 2005.

Olmstead, Taylor. *The Taming of Tina*. Penn State College of Medicine, Humanities, 2012. http://med.psu.edu/c/document_library/get_file?uuid=4a9b0a03-0c68-431a-85c3-5b63bdce4261&groupId=99092.

Pistorio, Ashley L. *Vita Perseverat*. Penn State College of Medicine, Humanities, 2010. http://med.psu.edu/c/document_library/get_file?folderId=2201894&name=DLFE-24805.pdf.

Powell, Nate. *Swallow Me Whole*. Marietta, GA: Top Shelf, 2008.

Satrapi, Marjane. *Embroideries*. New York: Pantheon Books, 2005.

———. *Persepolis*. 1st American ed. New York: Pantheon Books, 2003.

The Savage Sword of Conan the Barbarian. New York: Curtis Magazines [later Marvel Comics], 1974–95.

Schrag, Ariel. *Potential: The High School Chronicles of Ariel Schrag*. New York: Simon and Schuster, 2008.

Sendak, Maurice. *In the Night Kitchen*. New York: Harper and Row, 1970.

Shelton, Gilbert. *The Collected Adventures of the Fabulous Furry Freak Brothers*. San Francisco: Rip Off Press, 1971–92.

Siegel, Jerry, Joe Shuster, et al. *Superman* [later *The Adventures of Superman*]. Vol. 1. New York: DC Comics, 1938–86.

Sim, Dave. *Cerberus*. Ontario: Aardvark-Vanheim, 1977–2004.

Small, David. *Stitches*. New York: W. W. Norton, 2009.

Spiegelman, Art. *Maus*. New York: Pantheon Books, 1986.

Starr, Ann. "Where Babies Come From: A Miracle Explained." Artist book. 1997.

Stassen, Jean-Philippe. *Deogratias: A Tale of Rwanda*. Translated by Alex Siegel. 1st American ed. New York: First Second, 2006.

Tezuka, Osamu. *Ode to Kirihito*. Translated by Camellia Nieh. 1st American ed. New York: Vertical, 2006.

Tomorrow, Tom. "Immortality for Achievers." *The New Yorker*, July 2, 2001, 88.

Trudeau, Garry. *Doonesbury*. Syndicated, 1970–.

Weird War Tales. New York: DC Comics, 1971–83.

Wertz, Julia. *The Infinite Wait and Other Stories*. Toronto: Koyama, 2012.

Williams, Ian. *The Bad Doctor*. Hove, England: Myriad Editions, 2014.

Wynn, Kapit, and Lawrence M. Elson. *The Anatomy Coloring Book*. New York: Harper and Row, 1977.

Yang, Gene Luen. *American Born Chinese*. New York: First Second, 2006.

Yang, Gene Luen, and Thien Pham. *Level Up*. New York: First Second, 2011.

AUTHOR BIOGRAPHIES AND ACKNOWLEDGMENTS

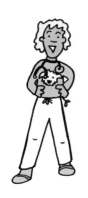

MK Czerwiec is Artist-in-Residence at Northwestern Feinberg School of Medicine. She has a B.A. in English from Loyola University of Chicago and a BSN from Rush University. Her M.A. is in medical humanities and bioethics from Northwestern, and her clinical nursing experience is in AIDS care and hospice care. MK has been making comics under the pseudonym Comic Nurse (http://www.comicnurse.com) since 2000. With Ian Williams she co-runs the Graphic Medicine website (http://www.graphicmedicine.org) and is on the organizing committee for the annual International Comics and Medicine conferences. MK also coordinates the Chicago chapter of London's salon, Laydeez Do Comics. She is currently creating her first graphic novel, the working title of which is *Taking Turns*. It will be an illustrated memoir/oral history of the AIDS unit in Chicago where she worked from 1994 to 2000. MK would like to thank all who helped to make this book a reality, including her colleagues at Penn State, Penn State University Press, and the Department of Medical Humanities and Bioethics at Northwestern University. She would also like to thank Cindy, for everything.

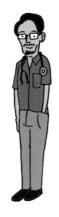

Ian Williams is a physician, comics artist, and writer based in Brighton, UK. He founded the Graphic Medicine website (http://www.graphicmedicine.org) in 2007 and currently edits it with MK Czerwiec. He has written book chapters and papers for various medical, humanities, and comics publications, and he chaired the organizing committee of the first Comics and Medicine conference in London in 2010. His graphic novel, *The Bad Doctor,* was published in June 2014 by Myriad Editions. He loves animals, riding bicycles, listening to melancholy music, and drinking tea. Ian would like to thank Kendra Boileau, Laura Jones, Krista Quesenberry, and Marc Zaffran, as well as his co-authors, Kimberly, Michael, MK, Scott, and Susan.

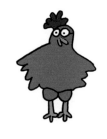

Susan Merrill Squier is thrilled to be a chicken in this volume, because chickens are the avatar of all humans: poor, forked, featherless beasts. A professor of women's studies and English at Penn State University, her affiliation with chickens explains her most recent book, *Poultry Science, Chicken Culture: A Partial Alphabet*. Her previous books include *Liminal Lives: Imagining The Human at the Frontiers of Biomedicine* and *Babies in Bottles: Twentieth-Century Visions of Reproductive Technology*. Susan thanks the graphic medicine collective, Kendra Boileau, Krista Quesenberry, Jarod Roselló, her students in the Penn State University Graphic Fiction and Graphic Medicine graduate seminars, and Gowen, Caitlin, and Toby.

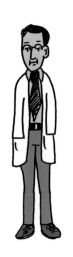

Michael J. Green is a physician, ethicist, researcher, and educator at Penn State College of Medicine, and he has been (along with collaborators on this book) a pioneer in using comics to teach medical students. He is professor of humanities and internal medicine, chair of the hospital ethics committee, and the author of numerous publications on end-of-life decision making, graphic medicine, and bioethics. Though depicted wearing a white coat and tie throughout this book, in real life, he almost never dresses like this. Michael would like to thank all those who helped bring this book to fruition, including family, colleagues, students, and friends who not only didn't laugh at the idea of teaching comics to medical students but provided encouragement and support for him to pursue this passion wherever it would lead.

author
biographies and
acknowledgments

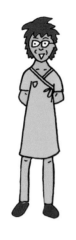

Kimberly R. Myers is delighted that MK and Ian finally gave her avatar a dye job back to dark hair, especially since she (the real Kimberly) worked super hard to get rid of that hot blond wig (double entendre) she wore for ten months! A professor of English by training—modern poetry and Irish literature are her first disciplinary loves—she now teaches medical students at Penn State College of Medicine, serving both as co-director of medical humanities and director of competency-based assessment and reflective learning. She also hosts the Penn State College of Medicine Physician Writers Group that she founded a few years back. Kimberly's great joy is working with dynamic, complex, and kind human beings of the student, colleague, and sometimes even chicken (!) variety, and she is especially grateful to be working with *this* creative lot. She is also deeply grateful to Dr. Pamela Wagar Smith for drawing what she was not yet ready to draw: to modify the words of James Joyce, "Me. And me then."

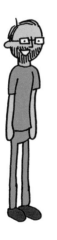

Scott T. Smith is an associate professor of English and comparative literature at Penn State University, where he teaches classes in medieval literature, early English language, and comics. He is especially interested in the broad circulation and use of comics and the ways in which comics acquire cultural value in different spaces. He is also interested in the legacy and diversity of comics as a global creative medium. His comics mantra: read more and read widely. Scott would like to thank Kendra Boileau, MK Czerwiec, Paul Gravett, Michael Green, Kimberly Myers, Krista Quesenberry, Jarod Roselló, Emily Smith, Susan Squier, and Ian Williams.

CREDITS

Chapter 2

Ruben Bolling, "Bad Blastocyst," from Bolling, *Thrilling Tom the Dancing Bug Stories: A Collection of the Weekly Comic Strip "Tom the Dancing Bug"* (Kansas City, MO: Andrews McMeel, 2004). Used by permission of Universal Uclick. All rights reserved.

Excerpts from Kaisa Leka, *I Am Not These Feet* (Helsinki: Absolute Truth Press, 2008), appear courtesy of Kaisa Leka.

Excerpts from Ann Starr, "Where Babies Come From: A Miracle Explained," appear courtesy of Ann Starr.

Chapter 3

Excerpt from Brian Fies, *Mom's Cancer* (New York: Abrams Image, 2006), appears courtesy of Brian Fies.

Graphic novel excerpts from *Cancer Vixen: A True Story*, by Marisa Acocella Marchetto, copyright © 2006 by Marisa Acocella Marchetto. Used by permission of Alfred A. Knopf, an imprint of the Knopf Doubleday Publishing Group, a division of Random House LLC. All rights reserved. Any third party use of this material, outside of this publication, is prohibited. Interested parties must apply directly to Random House LLC for permission.

Excerpts from Taylor Olmstead, *The Taming of Tina*, appear courtesy of Taylor Olmstead.

Excerpts from Julia Wertz, *The Infinite Wait and Other Stories* (Toronto: Koyama, 2012), are used by permission of Julia Wertz.

Chapter 4

The poem "Reconstruction," by Lisa Katz, was previously published in *Illness in the Academy*, edited by Kimberly R. Myers (West Lafayette: Purdue University Press, 2007). Used by permission.

Graphic novel excerpts from *Cancer Vixen: A True Story*, by Marisa Acocella Marchetto, copyright © 2006 by Marisa Acocella Marchetto. Used by permission of Alfred A. Knopf, an imprint of the Knopf Doubleday Publishing Group, a division of Random House LLC. All rights reserved. Any third party use of this material, outside of this publication, is prohibited. Interested parties must apply directly to Random House LLC for permission.

Comics by Pamela Wagar Smith appear courtesy of Pamela Wagar Smith.

Excerpts from Ashley L. Pistorio, *Vita Perseverat*, appear courtesy of Ashley Pistorio.

Chapter 5

Albrecht Dürer, *Melancholia I*. Image © Trustees of the British Museum.

Excerpt from Andrew Godfrey, *The CF Diaries* (Bristol: Sicker Than Thou Industries, 2011), appears courtesy of Andrew Godfrey.

Excerpts from Glyn Dillon, *The Nao of Brown* (London: Harry N. Abrams, 2012), appear courtesy of Glyn Dillon.

Chapter 6

Kathryn Fay, *My Summer Vacation*, appears courtesy of Kathryn Fay.

Comics by Muna Al-Jawad appear courtesy of Muna Al-Jawad.